P9-CPZ-369

Brooks – Cork Library
Shelton State
Community College

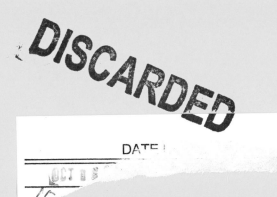

DATE

OCT

Memory
and Emotion

MAPS OF THE MIND
Steven Rose, General Editor

Pain: The Science of Suffering
Patrick Wall

The Making of Intelligence
Ken Richardson

How Brains Make up Their Minds
Walter J. Freeman

Sexing the Brain
Lesley Rogers

Intoxicating Minds: How Drugs Work
Ciaran Regan

How to Build a Mind: Toward Machines with Imagination
Igor Alexander

The Ageing Brain
Lawrence Whalley

The Unbalanced Mind
Julian Leff

Memories are Made of This: How Memory Works In Humans and Animals
Rusiko Bourtchouladze

DISCARDED

Memory
and Emotion

The Making of
Lasting Memories

James L. McGaugh

Brooks – Cork Library
Shelton State
Community College

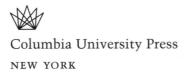

Columbia University Press

NEW YORK

Columbia University Press
Publishers Since 1893
New York   Chichester, West Sussex

Copyright © 2003 James L. McGaugh

All rights reserved

Library of Congress Cataloging-in-Publication Data

McGaugh, James L.
   Memory and emotion : preserving the presence of the past / James L. McGragh.
      p. cm. – (Maps of the mind)
   Includes bibliographical references and index.
   ISBN 0-231-12022-2 (alk. paper)
   1. Autobiographical memory. 2. Emotions. I. Title. II. Series.

BF378.A87M34 2003
153.1'2--dc21

                                                            2003051480

∞

Columbia University Press books are printed on permanent
and durable acid-free paper.

Printed in the United Kingdom

c 10 9 8 7 6 5 4 3 2 1

First published by Weidenfeld & Nicolson Ltd, London

To Becky

Contents

Preface

This book is about making and preserving memories. Memories are generally good things to have. Our records of our personal past are essential in enabling us to survive. All of our knowledge of our world, and our skills in living in it, are based on memories of our experiences. So, too, are all of our plans and dreams. Life without memory is difficult to imagine. After all, imagination requires memory. A life without memory would be no life at all.

Scientific studies of memory, started only a little over a century ago, have amply confirmed the conclusion that practice makes perfect. We all know that rehearsal of information or skills creates stronger memories. Much education is, of course, based on this general principle; but there is another way to make strong memories of experiences, and that is the central focus of this book. This other way has been long known but only recently the subject of scientific inquiry. In medieval times, before writing was used to keep historical records, other means had to be found to maintain records of important events, such as the granting of land to a township, an important wedding or negotiations between powerful families. To accomplish this, a young child about seven years old was selected, instructed to observe the proceedings carefully, and then thrown into a river. In this way, it was said, the memory of the event would be impressed on the child and the record of the event maintained for the child's lifetime.

Although I only recently learned about this medieval

memory aid, I have investigated neurobiological processes that underlie its effectiveness for almost half a century. My discussion of this topic is embedded in a larger context of the conditions affecting lasting memory in animals and humans. As much of the research on brain processes enabling memory investigates memory in animals, I discuss some of the critical findings revealing the complexity of animal memory. Their memory systems are much like our own, though the content of their memories doubtless differs in many ways from ours.

Research from many laboratories has revealed that there are different forms of memory that involve the actions of distinct brain systems; but there is also a promiscuous system that enabled the lasting memory of the medieval child thrown into the river. Emotional arousal activates stress hormones that, in turn, stimulate a specific brain system that regulates the consolidation of recently acquired information in other brain regions. A little stress is good for making lasting memories; but it is not always good to have strong, long-lasting memories. Fortunately, all memories are not created equal. Trivial and traumatic experiences should, and do, create memories that differ in durability. Experiences that induce intense emotional arousal can result in post-traumatic stress disorder. Furthermore, there is compelling evidence that individuals who have exceptionally strong memories can have exceptionally unsuccessful lives. Selectivity in creating memories is critically important. For most of us, built-in neurobiological systems automatically provide that needed selectivity. Our remembrance of experiences tends to vary directly with their emotional significance.

I have written this book for a general readership. It deals with questions about memory that I have been asked by family members, friends, neighbours and colleagues. Thus, I hope that anyone interested in the nature and bases of memory will find it to be informative and useful. On many occasions I have been asked what motivated me to write it. A simple answer is that Steven Rose asked me to write a book for the series 'Maps of the Mind', for which he is the editor. I thank Steven for inviting me to undertake this task. Another simple answer is that I found it easy to say yes, as I was intrigued by the challenge of writing a book on memory – especially emotion and memory – for the general public. It has provided me the opportunity of distilling my own almost half-century of research on memory consolidation and integrating it with findings from a great many other laboratories to discuss the actions of stress hormones and brain systems in creating lasting records of our personal pasts.

I want to thank my students and other research colleagues, past and present, for their very significant contributions to the findings and ideas discussed in the book. I thank Norm Weinberger, Larry Cahill, Ivan Izquierdo and Aryeh Routtenberg for their comments on sections of early drafts. I am grateful to Nancy Collett for patiently and carefully aiding the preparation of the many drafts of each chapter. Finally, I thank my wife Becky for her comments on early drafts of the chapters and for her sustained encouragement.

1 | **The Mystery of Memory**

I am standing backstage, closely watching my fellow actors in the play and waiting for the line that is a cue for my entry onstage. I hear the cue and am gripped by panic: I don't remember my lines in the play – not a single word. It is now too late for me to relearn them. I am to make my entrance onstage. All things considered, the best thing for me to do is to wake up so that I can leave the scene. So that is what I do. Each time this dream recurs I remain helplessly unprepared for my role in the play. The memory required for my entry onstage never appears.

This particular dream is a rather strange one. From childhood through graduate school I performed in many plays, bands and orchestras and always managed to learn and remember my parts: no memory failure. In my first years in college I studied drama and music. Perhaps it was there that the intense pressure of learning and remembering created its lasting influence that manages, even these days (or, rather, nights), to disturb my sleep and motivate my sustained interest in the workings of memory. There were always new lines to learn and even newer ones when scenes were rewritten during rehearsals. There were always new parts to learn, remember and, eventually, perform. Fortunately, unlike my dream experience, the memory required for the performances always managed to be there. Though curious, my dream conveys a serious message: memory is absolutely critical for our existence as humans. Without memory we can't plan to go onstage – or anywhere, for that matter – or even imagine doing so.

We are all, in some way, deeply interested in memory. Whether we want to know why we forget, how to improve our memory and prevent its decline or simply to understand what it is and how it works, memory is a topic that greatly concerns and intrigues us. Performers want to know why they get 'stage fright' and forget what it was that they were supposed to perform. Teachers and parents want to know how to improve learning and its product, memory, in children. Those who have had traumatic experiences long to forget them. The elderly and their family members worry about signs and consequences of diseases of memory. From time to time we all wonder about why it is that we forget where we placed our car keys or glasses and why it is that we know that we know something that we can't at the moment recall (but will, no doubt sometime later). The shelves of health-food stores bursting with herbal supplements claiming to increase brainpower and boost memory, provide striking testimony to our interest in and worry about memory. The intense competition among pharmaceutical and biotech companies to develop effective drugs for treating those with real (or imagined) declining memory is yet another sign of our very strong interest in and concern about it: we are willing to pay money for memory.

This is not surprising, as memory is very clearly worth paying for; it is, without doubt, our most important possession, our most critical capacity. We *are*, after all, our memories. It is our memory that enables us to value everything else we possess. Lacking memory, we would have no ability to be concerned about our hearts, hair, lungs, libido, loved ones, enemies, achievements, failures, incomes or income taxes. Our memory provides us with an autobiographical record and enables us to understand and react appropriately to changing experiences. Memory is the 'glue' of our personal existence. We live our lives moment by moment. The experiences of each immediately past moment are memories that, like individual frames of films that create moving pictures, merge with current momentary experiences to create the impression of seamless continuity in our lives – the integration of past, present and future.

Memory, in a most general sense, is the lasting consequence of an experience; but it is clearly more than that, as the same can be said for sunburn, blisters and calluses. More specifically, memory is the consequence of *learning* from an experience – that is, the consequence of acquiring new information. We learn and remember many kinds of information. We remember specific events in our lives, we remember facts without knowing when or where we learned them and we perform skills that we may not even know that we retain. For example, you remember what a bicycle is. You may remember your first bicycle and riding it as well, and perhaps falling off of it on a specific occasion. You may also remember how to ride a bicycle; and you will certainly remember that the words 'remember' and 'bicycle' appeared several times in recent sentences. Research is revealing the brain processes enabling these different kinds of remembrance: general knowledge, autobiographical memory of personal events, skills and recent memory.[1] These different forms of memory co-exist in our ordinary experiences and behaviour. While riding a bicycle (i.e. using the remembered skill) you can, of course, remember the word 'bicycle' and recall previous experiences with bicycles. You might also remember reading this section about remembering 'bicycle' experiences. Our brains have an amazing capacity to integrate the combined effects of our past experiences together with our present experiences in creating our thoughts and actions. How they manage to do this is one of the greatest scientific mysteries; but memory will not remain mysterious. The research findings discussed in this book clearly indicate that the veil of mystery is now being removed.

Not in the heavens

Memory, our most precious personal capacity, has been studied scientifically for just over a century. In contrast, the stars and planets quite distant from us have been studied for many centuries. Psychological science began its emergence from philosophy and physiology only in the latter part of the nineteenth century. In my later undergraduate years, as my interest in learning and memory deepened, I was a student in a Department of Philosophy and Psychology. I think that this department name continued to reflect a subtle but sustained scepticism that mental processes, such as memory, were a proper subject of scientific inquiry. It was perhaps thought better to keep such subjects in the realm of philosophy, or at least to hedge the bet. Studies of distant objects in the heavens no longer needed philosophical constraints. Astronomy was free to reject the prior conclusion that the Earth was the centre of the universe. Inquiring into the centre of human existence was, and to some extent remains, another matter entirely.

Psychological science was originally developed as the study of the content of the adult normal human mind. Introspection – that is, self-description of mental processes – was used for investigation and analysis. Critics argued, quite appropriately, that this approach was doomed by the lack of objectivity, a cardinal criterion for scientific analysis, and that descriptive analysis did not lead to experimental investigation. The critics were correct, of course. A purely subjective method of introspection is clearly unsuitable for a scientific study of memory. Without some means of objective verification, how is it possible for you to know whether my assertions about my personal memories are valid? You would certainly question the validity of my memory were I simply to assert that I remember (i.e. introspectively recall) hearing Lincoln deliver his Gettysburg Address or that I can recall all of Shakespeare's plays, word for word (or measure for measure). You would, I presume, even question whether I remember any of the lines I learned for plays when I was a college student. As we all know, and as I discuss more extensively later in this book, our memories are not perfect; they are fallible. There is more than a little justification for the saying, 'Of all liars, the smoothest and most convincing is memory.' Thus, objective analysis is required, for study of memory, even as it is for study of the heavens. Fortunately, there are objective ways of finding out whether I remember what I claim to remember, just as there are objective ways to study the distant planets and stars in the heaven.

How to get to Carnegie Hall

'I have been here but a little while but have come, full of devotion, to meet and know a man of whom the world speaks with such reverence.'

This is a line that I remember from a part that I had in the play *Faust* when I was a freshman in college. The accuracy of my memory of that line could, of course, be checked by reading the play – that is one way to study memory objectively; but, maybe it is not actually a line in the play after all. If accurate (and I confess that I have not checked to determine whether it is), it would provide some evidence that information well learned is well remembered; but that would be weak evidence, at best. The pioneering studies by the German psychologist Hermann Ebbinghaus published in 1885[2] were the first to show us what was needed to demonstrate that memory can be investigated objectively by experimental study. Ebbinghaus studied learning and memory using himself as the subject. He introduced the use of 'nonsense syllables' – three-letter consonant–vowel–consonant syllables that were not German words – to minimize the effect of familiarity with the material to be learned. He memorized lists of syllables by repeating them until he learned them, as he said, 'by heart'. At a later time he then tested his memory by measuring the decrease in repetitions required to relearn the lists.

As anyone offering advice about how to get to Carnegie Hall knows, learning detailed and precise complex information and skills well requires practice, practice, practice. Ebbinghaus could certainly have offered that advice, as he found that poorly learned material is very rapidly forgotten. However, he also found that increases in strength of learning increase the strength of memory tested the next day and that repeated daily relearning greatly improves memory on each subsequent day. Although these are now not particularly surprising findings, they were highly important ones for both scientific and practical reasons. Ebbinghaus's findings laid to rest the widely held view that mental functions such as memory could not be studied by objective experimental research. His pioneering research created the cornerstone for memory research. It also greatly influenced early research investigating effective procedures in education. It should be no surprise that 'cramming' for an examination is an ineffective way of learning. This information alone is important for anyone wanting to remember better. In terms of its scientific basis, Ebbinghaus's conclusions offer advice that is vastly superior to the dubious claims on labels of herbal supplements on health-food shelves. Why should we expect to have strong memories of things we learn poorly? Most of us who claim that we have a 'poor memory' are simply offering a poor excuse.

A word about Ebbinghaus's statement that he 'learned by heart'. Of course we know now, as he no doubt knew then, that he learned 'by brain' and not 'by heart'. He can be excused for using the words 'by heart', because although almost four centuries have passed since Harvey showed that the heart is merely a pump for circulating blood, we still use that curious expression derived from an ancient, flawed hypothesis about the anatomy of memory. As there is much that we do not yet understand about memory, we no doubt also have modern flawed hypotheses about brain and memory that will subsequently be discarded only by careful research and scientific consensus.

Brooks – Cork Library
Shelton State
Community College

Significance and remembrance

'I remember seeing bits of wing and fuselage bobbing like toys on a churning surface. I remember seeing scraps of luggage and clothing. And I remember seeing bodies, torn and mutilated beyond description. Calamity has a way of imprinting itself on memory.'[3]

Although repetition is a highly effective way of making strong, long-lasting memories, it is not the only way. For better or for worse (and it can be both), highly arousing emotional experiences are also well remembered. The remembrances quoted above refer to a plane crash that occurred many decades earlier. It seems highly unlikely that the person quoted remembers equally well, if at all, the events of a day in the weeks before or after witnessing the crash scene. We all have lasting memories of emotionally arousing experiences. Intense emotional arousal such as that induced by witnessing an air-crash scene is not required. We remember both pleasant and unpleasant experiences. Certainly, lottery winners and Nobel Prize winners remember where they were and what they were doing when they learned the good news. We tend to remember praises and embarrassments, successes and disappointments, weddings and divorces, births and deaths, birthdays and holidays and significant news events; for an American, 911 is no longer simply a phone number to call in the event of an emergency. The events of September 11, 2001 created memories that may last a lifetime in millions of people throughout the world. Such memories clearly are not among those that fade quickly.

Why do some, perhaps most, memories fade, whereas memories of other unique experiences are preserved? Why is it that memories of emotionally arousing experiences are favoured? This is a central question addressed in this book, but in asking it we must also look (as with all questions of memory) for evidence that these favoured memories are accurate. Claiming that they are does not, of course, constitute proof that they are: evidence is required; and reasonably possible alternative explanations for the strength of this kind of memory need to be considered carefully. For example, as emotionally intense experiences are typically recalled often, the possibility that repeated rehearsal of the experiences may influence the durability of the memories cannot easily be excluded – that is, there may be an 'Ebbinghaus' effect even for such unique experiences. However, as I discuss later in the book, there is considerable evidence indicating that emotionally arousing experiences do not need to be rehearsed in order to be well remembered; but such experiences do need to be remembered. There is an enormous adaptive value in being able to remember emotionally significant events: dangerous and disgusting situations need to be avoided; memories of successful experiences help create future successes. Fortunately for us and the other animals, this adaptive function is provided automatically by hormonal and brain systems activated by emotional experiences. Knowledge of Ebbinghaus is not needed for this adaptive influence.

Despite the considerable and critical influence of repetition and emotional activation on the formation of our memories, forgetting of ordinary experiences of daily life is usually inevitable; and although we don't usually think of it in this way, the ability to forget is also important. Most memories are not cherished. We usually don't need to remember where we placed our car keys one day last month, or what we had for breakfast last Tuesday; and, ordinarily, we do not: memories of the trivia of our lives generally fade quickly. Although memories of extremely traumatic experiences such as witnessing the scene of a plane crash are strong and long-lasting, they are usually not indelible in detail; and for perhaps most such experiences it is good that memories are not indelible. The 'imprinting' effects of calamity, like those of ordinary daily experiences, typically fade somewhat over time; but for horrific traumatic memories, the time required for evidence of fading may be many months, years or decades.

As most of what we know about how neurobiological systems create memories has come from studies of memory in animals, it is essential, first, to consider how memory is studied in animals. We need to know how we discover what animals 'know' about their previous experiences. The effort is complicated (but made more interesting) by the fact that there are several forms of memory and that, as memory is not directly observed but inferred from behaviour, it is not easy to get animals to tell us the truth about what they remember – or what they forget. I turn now to that important issue.

2 | Dogs, Cats, Chimps and Rats: Habits and Memory

Our memories exist in different forms. In his highly engaging and enormously influential book *The Principles of Psychology*, published in 1890,[1] William James was the first to propose that there are different forms of memory. His insights into various forms of memory remain the focus of much memory research even today. He distinguished between 'primary memory' for memory immediately following an experience, and 'memory proper', or 'secondary memory', for the later recall of the experience. Today the terms 'short-term memory' and 'working memory' refer to memory for recent experiences, and 'long-term memory' refers to lasting explicit memory of specific events (episodic memory) or explicit general knowledge of facts (semantic memory).[2] Interestingly, James discussed *habits*, the memorial products of extensive practice that he regarded as mere learned reflexes, in an earlier, separate chapter of his book. He wrote: 'When we look at living creatures...one of the first things that strike us is that they are bundles of habits...In action grown habitual, what instigates each new muscular contraction to take place in its appointed order is not a thought or a perception, but the sensation occasioned by the muscular contraction just finished.'[3]

Anyone who has learned to type, ski or to drive a car knows that, in a general sense, James was at least partly correct. Complex actions that at first require explicit memory of what just happened and a plan for what to do next eventually, with considerable practice, become relatively effortless and are performed reasonably well while we are thinking about other matters and doing other things. Certainly, as we know, many drivers eat, talk on mobile phones, manage unruly children and sometimes even read while driving on motorways. On the motorway, reasonably well is, of course, not good enough.

Habits (and forgotten memory) in dogs and cats

Habits, of course, require memory, but they differ from other forms of memory. Efforts to understand the way or ways in which habits and other forms of memory differ and the bases of their differences are the intense focus of much current memory research. However, the end of the nineteenth century marked the beginning of a converging effort to treat *all* learning as a reflex or habit. Memory was largely (but not completely, as I discuss later) forgotten, ignored or disdained for the next half-century. Even in the 1960s I was admonished by a journal editor to substitute the word 'retention' for 'memory' in a paper that I submitted for publication because the term 'memory' was considered to be too mentalistic and thus unsuitable for a scientific publication. Although the use of the term 'memory' was gradually re-emerging, at that time it still suffered from some sort of mild Victorian shame.

In order to understand current research on memory it is essential to know at least a bit of history. It all started with dogs and cats. The Russian physiologist I. P. Pavlov began his studies of 'classical conditioning' in dogs at the end of the nineteenth century.[4] At that same time the American psychologist E. L. Thorndike (a student of William James) began his studies of 'instrumental' habit learning in cats.[5] Why did these researchers, and many to follow, turn to animals to learn about learning? In nineteenth-century Russia, studies of physiology grew out of a rich tradition of research and theory concerning reflexes. For Pavlov, who was trained in this tradition, research

on conditioned reflexes in dogs was a natural consequence of
his prior studies of reflexive digestive processes, for which he
won the Nobel Prize. Very different reasons motivated the
research on animal learning in the United States. The lingering
ghosts of nineteenth-century introspective mentalism needed
to be exorcized. The study of behaviour, which came to be
known as 'behaviorism', and the use of animals as experimental subjects provided, it seemed at the time, the means to do
just that. After all, although you can ask your dog or cat to tell
you what it remembers, you certainly can't expect to get a
direct answer; but, by using purely behavioural responses, the
learning and retention of learned behaviour (note that I did not
use the word 'memory') can be studied objectively. For 'behaviorism', the fact that cats and dogs *can't* talk was helpful, if
not essential, in preventing mentalistic or anthropomorphic
contamination. A sceptic might say that this was perhaps a bit
like turning the lights off in order to avoid the possibility of
finding something interesting with the lights on. Even though
Ebbinghaus had already shown that learning and memory can
be studied objectively (that is, without reference to consciousness) in human subjects, animal learning studies quickly moved
to centre stage at the beginning of the twentieth century.
Pavlovian and Thorndikian approaches to learning were very
rapidly accepted and firmly established. As I discuss later, this
was in some ways fortunate, as laboratory animals are used
extensively in studies investigating the neurobiology of learning and memory and many current experiments use training
procedures such as those pioneered by Pavlov and Thorndike.

Though they were similar in the use of objective measures of
learning, the approaches, procedures and theoretical interpretations offered by Pavlov and Thorndike differed greatly. Pavlov's
procedures are so well known that they are very often depicted
in cartoons; but such cartoons do not, of course, accurately
reflect either the experimental procedures or the essential characteristics of the findings: cartoons are, after all, cartoons. In a
typical experiment by Pavlov, a dog restrained in a harness was

presented with a stimulus, such as a black square, followed by presentation of food powder. The food elicited the unlearned, or 'unconditioned', response of salivation. After a few pairings the previously neutral stimulus became a 'conditioned stimulus', or a signal for food – the 'unconditioned stimulus'. Thus, through the association of the two stimuli, the dog came to salivate when the black square was presented. Quite clearly, the dog's responses indicated that it had learned that one stimulus signalled another stimulus. One of Pavlov's assistants (Snarsky) initially interpreted such findings as evidence of the dogs' '...psychical activity, and...suggested taking into account the thoughts, desires and emotions of the animals. [He] stubbornly insisted on his subjective anthropomorphic interpretations of phenomena and finally had to leave Pavlov's laboratory.'[6]

Unfortunately for Snarsky (and perhaps for us as well), Pavlov came to a very different conclusion. Pavlov considered the conditioned reflex to be...

> ...what we recognize in ourselves and in animals under such names as training, discipline, education, habits; these are nothing but connections established in the course of individual existence, connections between definite external stimuli and corresponding reactions. Thus, the conditioned reflex opens to the physiologist the door to investigation of a considerable part, and possibly, of the entire nervous activity.[7]

We now know that Pavlov's view that conditioning is simply habit formation was oversimplified. Frankly, as we shall see, it was wrong. However, its influence on past as well as current learning theory and research cannot be overstated. Furthermore, Pavlov's view that the conditioned reflex would enable investigation of the nervous system, especially neural processes involved in learning, has been amply confirmed.

Those of us who are owned by cats may find it difficult to imagine using Pavlov's procedures to train cats. They are as suitable for restraint in a harness as they are for herding. Thus, it is not surprising that Thorndike used different training procedures from those used by Pavlov. Thorndike trained cats by placing a bowl of milk adjacent to their cage and allowing them to escape from the cage and get to the milk only by making a specific response, such as pressing on a latch or pulling on a string. As the cat's response was instrumental in obtaining the reward, the training procedure came to be known as 'instrumental learning'. Thorndike interpreted his findings as indicating that the *consequences* of the correct response, i.e. the reward, acted directly and automatically to strengthen the connection between the stimulus situation and a randomly emitted response – that is, he concluded that rewards created habits by strengthening stimulus-response (S-R) connections. Thorndike called this the 'law of effect'. Thorndike's findings and conclusions, which were known to Pavlov, contrasted with Pavlov's conclusions that conditioning results from the association between stimuli (i.e. S-S learning) and that the role of the reward (e.g. food) is to elicit the unconditioned response (e.g. salivation); but, for both, training created habits. Although neither stated it precisely in this way, for both Pavlov and Thorndike the habit *was* the memory of the training. Unlike James, Pavlov and Thorndike did not write separate chapters on 'memory' as, from their theoretical perspectives, none was required. Memory vanished. Habits were sufficient to account for learning.

Supposing for a moment that simple learned behaviour might, in fact, consist of reflex habits. What about learning (most learning, no doubt) that appears to be more complex than a simple reflex? At the very extreme, the American psychologist John B. Watson proposed that complex habits consist simply of chains of simple reflexes.[8] He suggested, for example, that thinking is merely implicit speech that can be analysed by studying the muscles of the larynx. Although this would seem to pose a major problem, to say the least, for memories that do not consist of speech or cannot be expressed in words (not to mention the critical and complex issue of syntax), that problem did not significantly restrain the considerable enthusiasm for Watsonian behaviourism at that time; but the sceptics – and there were many – referred to Watson's theory as 'muscle twitchism'.[9]

Habits as units of learning subsequently found their zenith in the enormously influential work of Clark Hull. His book *Principles of Behavior* (1943)[10] summarized his several decades of research (primarily on habit learning in rats) and presented them in a formal theory. It was not a modest undertaking. In the preface he wrote,

> ... this book attempts to present...the primary, or fundamental, molar principles of behavior. It has been written on the assumption that all behavior, individual and social, moral and immoral, normal and psychopathic, is generated from the same primary laws; that the differences in the objective behavioral manifestations are due to the differing conditions under which habits are set up and function.[11]

Hull's book was intended to be, as a chapter subheading indicated, 'A suggested prophylaxis against anthropomorphic subjectivism'.[12] From Hull's perspective, the real or imagined nineteenth-century ghosts had not yet been exorcized and he saw it as his responsibility to finish that task. In essence, Hull's theory combined the views of Pavlov and Thorndike in proposing that S-R habits are based on the reinforcing effects of rewards (i.e. the 'law of effect'); and all learned behaviour was thought to consist of such S-R habits. Hull's theory had no need or room for the concept of memory.

Memory remembered in chimps and rats

Do S-R habits provide a sufficient explanation of learned behaviour? In the mid-1950s, graduate students in the Department of Psychology at the University of California, Berkeley, produced each year a musical comedy parodying contemporary theory. One memorable (to me, at least) product of our efforts was a song, sung to the tune of, 'I've been working on the railroad', that went something like this:

> I believe in S-R theory things that I can see.
> Stimuli and their responses are quite enough for me.
> Let's forget about perception, memory won't be missed.
> If it can't be said in S-R, it does not exist.

Although S-R theory enjoyed wide acceptance for several decades, it was increasingly challenged by a host of very embarrassing findings – findings, that is, that did not fit the theory at all. At the peak of Pavlov's and Thorndike's influence the German psychologist Wolfgang Köhler saw no evidence of trial-and-error habit learning in his studies of learning in chimpanzees;[13] rather, he saw evidence of insightful learning. When placed in a cage with boxes strewn around the floor and a banana hanging from the top of the cage, chimps gathered the boxes and stacked them in an effort to reach the banana. When sticks were strewn about the floor and the banana was placed outside the cage, the chimps tried to retrieve the banana with the sticks and even tried to put sticks together in order to reach bananas placed beyond the reach of a single stick. The animals appeared to learn by grasping the relationships between objects and using the information (i.e. memory) to solve problems – in clear violation of the 'law of effect': the learning occurred *before* the reward was obtained.

Additionally, increasing evidence revealed that Pavlovian and instrumentally conditioned responses are not simply habits based on reflexes. For example, Karl Lashley, a pioneering investigator of brain processes and memory (and, most interestingly, John B. Watson's student), conducted a direct and devastating test of Watson's theory that complex learning is based on chains of conditioned reflexes.[14] Lashley trained rats in a maze and then induced a large lesion in each rat's cerebellum, a brain region known to be important for control of movements. Although the brain damage severely disrupted the rats' ability to walk, it did not destroy their memory of the maze. The rats managed to wobble and, in some cases, tumble down the correct maze pathway. Clearly, the rats' maze learning could not have consisted simply of S-R reflex chains.

The view that Pavlovian conditioning consists simply of a learned reflex was also challenged by many experiments. In most experiments in Pavlov's laboratory, dogs were 'conditioned' and tested while restrained in a harness. On one occasion a dog that had been trained with food (with salivation as the response) was released from the harness. When the conditioning signal was presented, 'The dog at once ran to the machine, wagged its tail at it, tried to jump up to it, barked, and so on; in other words, it showed as clearly as possible the whole system of behavior patterns serving... to beg [for] food... It is, in fact this whole system that is being conditioned in the classical experiment.'[15]

In another classical conditioning experiment (this one not conducted in Pavlov's laboratory), a well-trained sheep restrained in a harness flexed its leg when a signal previously paired with leg shock was presented. However – and most interestingly – the sheep made a very different response when it was placed on its back and the signal presented: '...flexion of the foreleg fails to occur; instead all four limbs are stiffened and the animal attempts to lift its head'.[16] It certainly seems appropriate to ask what happened to the sheep's well-established 'reflex habit'. The habit vanished but the sheep's memory of the significance of the signal did not.

Starting in the 1920s and continuing into the 1950s, the American psychologist Edward Tolman mounted the major insurrection against S-R habit learning theory. Tolman saw very little, if any, evidence of reflex habit learning. In his book with the provocative title *Purposive Behavior in Animals and Men* (1932) (see reference 9), he observed that even rats acquire explicit knowledge (i.e. cognition) that can be used flexibly (rather than reflexively) and in a purposive way. He, too, was a behaviourist with a strong anti-introspectionistic bias. Cognition and purpose were not derived from anthropomorphic introspection

but, rather, were *inferred* from objective observation of the rats'
behaviour. He argued that the analysis of learned behaviour
should focus on what he called 'molar acts', not on reflexes. In
Tolman's own words:

> A rat running a maze; a cat getting out of a puzzle box; a man driving
> home to dinner; a child hiding from a stranger... a psychologist recit-
> ing a list of nonsense syllables... – These are behaviors... And it
> must be noted that in mentioning no one of them have we referred
> to, or, we blush to confess it, for the most part even known, what
> were the exact muscles and glands, sensory nerves, and motor nerves
> involved.[17]

In a direct challenge to S-R views of learning Tolman and his
students demonstrated that maze learning does not require
rewards. In a classic study of what he termed 'latent learning',
rats given an unrewarded trial in a maze each day for several
days did not reduce their errors (entries of blind alleys) – that is,
their performance gave no evidence of learning. However, the
rats clearly learned and remembered information about the
maze acquired on the early non-rewarded training trials.
Subsequently, when daily trials in the maze were rewarded by
food, the rats' performance improved immediately and was
comparable to that of rats given a reward on each daily training
trial. These findings violated the 'law of effect' and led, ultimately (that is, after several decades), to its rejection and the
demise of Hullian influences. Although rewards may influence
what we and the other animals do, it is now abundantly clear
that they do not act by automatically strengthening S-R connections. Thus, the 'law of effect' now belongs in the
Smithsonian Institution alongside other interesting but failed
historical relics such as tubas played with oboe-reed mouth-
pieces. It certainly does not belong in any modern theory of
learning and memory.

Thinking and theory about the nature and causes of behaviour in the late nineteenth and early twentieth centuries were

heavily influenced by contemporary developments in other areas of culture, science and technology. Puppets and mechanical toys (automata) preset to perform specific actions were common. The telegraph and telephone enabled communication by means of specific connections and reconnections of wires. The course of a cannonball fired into the air was determined by prior calculations. Hull, for example, suggested that it was helpful to consider '... the behaving organism as a completely self-maintaining robot, constructed of materials as unlike ourselves as may be, [and]... to consider the various general problems in behavior dynamics which must be solved in the design of a truly self-maintaining robot'.[18] The notion of a purposive, goal-directed machine was – well, unthinkable. Today it is not. We are surrounded by devices that are purposive in the sense that they vary their activity relative to some set point. Today our missiles are guided. Computers, which were, paradoxically, originally developed to compute ballistic trajectories, are almost unlimited in their ability to enable our modern devices to respond flexibly to changing circumstances and with reference to specific outcomes. If machines can act purposively, certainly there should be no problem in concluding that dogs, cats, chimpanzees and humans can do so as well. The ability to behave purposively clearly requires memory: habits won't do the job.

At this point I have to confess that I was a student of Tolman (sometimes referred to as a 'Tolmanian' or, on occasion a 'Tolmaniac') and served as his teaching assistant. As a very proper New Englander, he was both fair and restrained in his class discussions of other contemporary views of learning; but in one lecture commenting on the limitations of S-R theory he pointed out that, as there are important cognitive processes in the organism that intervene between the S and the R, at the very least, an 'O' (for 'organism') must be inserted. Moreover, as it is behavioural acts that occur and not muscle-twitch responses, the 'R' should be changed to 'B' for 'behaviour'. He then, with a sly grin (and no doubt with some residual New England guilt), referred to S-R theory as the 'SOB' theory.

Pavlov is usually linked with Thorndike in discussions of learning because of his view of learning as consisting of reflex habits; but, in retrospect, it is more appropriate to link Pavlov with Tolman, for Tolman, like Pavlov, argued that learning consists of the formation of associations between stimuli, or S-S learning – again, in Tolman's terms, learning about 'what-leads-to-what'. The still widely promoted and popular view of Pavlovian conditioning is that a neutral stimulus, after pairing with an unconditioned stimulus – i.e. a stimulus that already elicits a particular response – will elicit the same response; but as the title of a paper by Robert Rescorla indicates: 'Pavlovian Conditioning. It's not what you think it is'. Conditioning does not consist simply of the shifting of a response from one stimulus to another or simply of learning the relationship between a neutral event and a valuable event. It is '...the learning that results from exposure to relation among events in the environment. Such learning is the primary means by which the organism represents the structure of its world.'[19]

The findings of an interesting experiment conducted by Michael Davis and his colleagues[20] investigating 'fear-potentiated startle' clearly illustrate the predictive consequences of Pavlovian conditioning. Rats first learned that a light signalled danger: a light was followed by footshock delivered to different groups, at delays varying from a few milliseconds to just under a minute. A few days later the light was presented (with no shock) and then, after a delay, a loud tone was presented and the animals' startle response to the tone was recorded. In all groups, the tone elicited startle. However, for the different groups, the degree of startle was greatest when the tone was presented at the light–shock delay interval that the rat had previously experienced. Remarkably, with but a single pairing of the light with footshock delivered after a delay of about a minute, the magnitude of the animals' startle was greatest when the tone was presented at that *same* delay after the light onset. The rats clearly learned not only *that* the light predicted footshock (what led to what); they also learned *when* to expect the footshock. Thus, they remembered a great deal about the relationships between events after but a single experience with them. Additionally, studies of 'sensory preconditioning' have shown that stimuli or events being associated do not have to be of any particular significance. If a light is associated with a tone, and the light is then used as a signal in a conditioning experiment, the tone will also subsequently elicit the conditioned response. A simple pairing of the light and tone a few times is sufficient for such learning.

Of course, as we all know, learning does not require specific training. Much learning occurs simply by observation. Certainly, children learn by observing. Lower animals also learn by observation, as is acknowleged by the expression, 'Monkey see, monkey do.' That conclusion has been confirmed by many experimental studies of observational learning in rats, cats and monkeys. Our representations of the world consist of our memories. Whether we receive specific training or simply learn by observing, our experience that certain events follow others leads us to expect or predict events (again, Tolman's 'what leads to what'). The smell of coffee predicts its taste and, perhaps, breakfast. The sound of a popping cork may predict the taste of champagne bubbles and a celebration. The sight of flashing blue or red lights in our rear-view mirror predicts a less pleasant outcome. Our response to each event depends upon what we expect or predict; and that, of course, is based on our memories of past events.

Memory and habit reconsidered

The evidence that dogs, cats, chimps, rats and human beings learn and remember complex relationships between events does not mean that they don't learn habits. They do, of course; and, as I discuss below, habits and explicit memory, or 'memory proper', to use William James's term, are acquired at the same time. First, however, we need to consider what might be meant by the term 'habit'.

I have the habits of using a computer, wearing shoes and driving a car. I also have the habits of eating three meals a day and sleeping at night. None of these statements refers to any highly specific learned and remembered movements. They are certainly not S-R habits; they are simply things I tend to do. Now it gets tricky. I also have the habit of playing the clarinet. Here the word 'habit' may have two very different meanings. First, I have a habit of playing the clarinet occasionally. Second, when I do so, I play it in very particular ways. Although my responses (breathing, blowing, moving my arms, hands and fingers) vary from moment to moment with the music being played, the sequences of responses used are based on what I previously learned from previous practice. I also have, of course, explicit memory of the music I am playing. The memory of the music being played consists of the learned and remembered *flexible* skill – not of highly specific discrete motor responses.

Most of us who have the habit of using computer keyboards type in very particular ways that may not even be known or remembered explicitly. Which finger, for example do you use to type 'o' or 'v'? Which fingers are used and in what order to type the words 'habit' and 'memory'? Although these are learned and remembered habitual responses, they remain highly flexible. After all, your typing of 'o' or 'v' is not constrained by the letter that precedes it; and the different movements made in typing each of these letters depend on the movements required by letters just typed. Thus, even the skill of typing is a highly flexible skill not to be explained by the acquisition of highly specific S-R reflex habits: William James was wrong. But again, your memory for a skill such as typing clearly differs from your memory *about* typing and your memory *that* you can type. So, if we are to use the term 'habit', it is important to be clear about the way in which we use the term. Specifically, we need to distinguish between the learned tendency to do something and the learned flexible skill used in doing it. Additionally, although very extensive training can result in the learning of a specific, precise, relatively simple motor movement, such as blinking the eyelid

in response to a brief signal,[21] this particular type of 'habit' learning, though important, is doubtless the exception, not the rule.
Furthermore, as we saw in the results of the Pavlovian conditioning studies discussed briefly above, the learning occurring with
such conditioning does not consist *of* the motor movement.
Other information is also acquired during the training. What
other information? You need to ask the subject that question in
order to find out.

Discovering 'what' is learned and remembered

Earlier in this chapter I wrote, '...although you can ask your dog
or cat to tell you what it remembers, you certainly can't expect
to get a *direct* answer'; but you *can* get an answer if you ask the
question in the right way. It is critically important to distinguish between the *methods used* to train animals and the
outcome of the training. Years ago my wife and I had a dog that
barked whenever the fence gate to the courtyard at the front of
our house was opened. As the barking often disturbed our
napping child (which, in turn, greatly disturbed the parents!), I
decided to teach the dog to be quiet when the gate opened by
slapping him lightly with a newspaper as he started to bark.
The long-term unsatisfactory outcome of this effort was that I
taught the dog to bark with his mouth shut while he hid behind
the piano.

There are, of course, many much better designed and more
informative studies investigating what animals 'know' after
they have been trained. The study by Michael Davis, discussed
above, showing that rats learn both *that* light predicts shock
and *when* the shock occurs after the light onset, is an excellent
example. Another very clever study, by Lawrence and di
Rivera,[22] asked if rats can learn the significance of the relationship between cues. On each of many training trials rats were
presented with a card painted a different shade of grey at the
upper and lower parts of the card. One of the shades of grey, a
medium grey, was always at the bottom of the card. Think of a

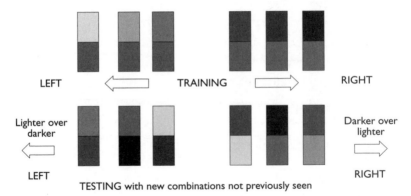

Figure 1A Learning about the relationships between stimuli. Rats were first trained with a series of cards having different shades of grey at the upper and lower parts of the card. The lower part was always a medium grey. They were rewarded for going left when the tops of the cards were lighter and going right when the tops of the cards were darker. They were then tested with new cards that had different shades of grey on the upper and lower parts. On most of the test trials the animals went left when the top of the card was lighter than the bottom and went right when the top of the card was darker. These findings indicate that the animals had learned to respond to the relationship between the top and bottom shades of grey. From Lawrence and di Rivera, 1954.

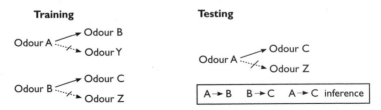

Figure 1B Learning to infer relationships between stimuli. Rats first learned to associate odour A with odour B and then to associate odour B with odour C. When subsequently tested with odour A, they chose odour C rather than another odour. The prior associations enabled the rats to infer that odour A was associated with odour C. From Bunsey and Eichenbaum, 1966.

medium grey as a '4', with '1' as a very light grey and '7' as a very dark grey. They were trained to turn in one direction, e.g. left, when light-grey shades 1, 2 or 3 appeared at the top of the card and to turn in the other direction, e.g. right, when dark shades 5, 6 or 7 appeared at the top (see figure 1A). It is possible that the rats might have learned six different responses: one to each of the cards; but subsequent tests asking the rats what they had learned yielded a very different answer: the rats learned and remembered that the critical cue was the *relationship* between the shades of grey at the top and bottom of the cards. They learned to turn left when the top card was lighter than the bottom card and to turn right when the top card was darker than the bottom card. For example, they turned left when presented with a shade 5 over a shade 7 (i.e. lighter over darker) on the test and turned right when shade 3 appeared over shade 1 (i.e. darker over lighter).

We cannot discover what an animal (or human subject, for that matter) has learned simply by knowing the specific training methods used. If we want to know what an animal knows, we have to ask it the right question. In the experiment just described, the experimenter asked the animals if they remembered that the relative brightness of the top and bottom of the card was the best cue to use in making a response; and the answer was yes, they did.

Rats' memories also enable them to make inferences about the significance of cues. In an ingenious set of experiments Howard Eichenbaum and his colleagues[23] trained rats to dig in a small container containing sand and a buried cereal reward. They were then trained to sample the distinctive odour (e.g. cinnamon, coffee etc.) of one container and choose one of two other containers with other distinctive odours (e.g. lemon, clove etc.), one of which always contained a cereal reward (see figure 1B). Using these procedures, the rats first learned to associate odour A with odour B rather than with another odour, Y. They then learned to associate odour B with odour C rather than with another odour, Z. Then came the critical test: the experimenters presented odour A as the sample and allowed the rats to choose between odour C and odour Z. As odour A had not been previously associated with either odour C or odour Z the responses on the test could not be predicted by prior direct

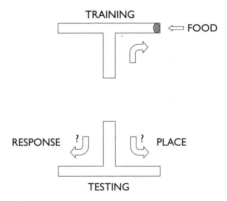

Figure 2 Rats readily learn to go to places in an apparatus (and room) where they are rewarded. Rats were first trained to find food in one alley of a T-maze (top of figure). The position of the maze was then rotated 180 degrees and the animals were tested to determine whether they had learned to make a right-turning response or to go to a location in the room. On the test, most animals did not make a right-turning response but, rather, turned left and went to the place where food had been found.

associations between the odours; but, that did not prevent the rats from correctly selecting odour C on the test. The association of A with B and B with C enabled the animals to *infer* that A was associated with C. These findings provide yet another problem for an S-R view of learning: the cue–reward associations acquired during training cannot account for the animals' responses on the test trial; inference based on memory is required.

Remembering where to go and what to do

The question 'What is learned' has also been asked in much less complex experiments. One simple apparatus, a T-shaped maze, was used as a major battleground in the intense fights between Hullian and Tolmanian forces in the middle of the past century. Studies of rats' learning in a T-maze were to settle the issue of whether the animals learned S-R responses or information about 'what leads to what'. In a typical experiment rats were placed in the starting alley and allowed to go left or right at the top of the T. Food was always placed at the same end of the top alley – for example, the right end (see figure 2). What did the animals learn from the training? Did they learn to make a turning response (S-R habit based on the law of effect), or did they learn about the place in the maze where food was found? To find out, the alley containing the food was left in place but the starting arm was placed on the other side, so that if the animals were originally trained to go north, they now started from the north and ran to the south. If they had learned a turning response, they would be expected to turn to the *right*, as they had in the original training, and enter the alley that had never contained food. If they had learned the location of food in the room they would be expected to turn *left* – i.e. make a response that was different from that made during the original training. In support of the Tolman view, most studies using these procedures found that the animals on the test trial chose to go to the place where food had been found before, despite the fact that it required them to make a different turning response from that made in the training.

However, as with most battles, it was not a clear-cut victory for the Tolmanians. Under some conditions the animals made the same turning response on the test trial as they had made during the previous training. One might conclude that both sides won – or that both lost. From the point of view of Hullian S-R theory, place learning was not possible. All learning was supposed to consist of S-R habits and there was no place in the theory for memory of the location of food. Tolman decided that there was, after all, room for the learning of responses – as long as they were behavioural acts such as turning and not muscle-twitch responses – and published an ecumenical paper entitled: 'There is More Than One Kind of Learning';[24] but that paper did not explain why it is that animals sometimes learn to make responses (again, behavioural acts, not specific motor contractions) even though they are quite capable of remembering the place where food is found. It was a concession, not a satisfactory resolution of the theoretical conflict.

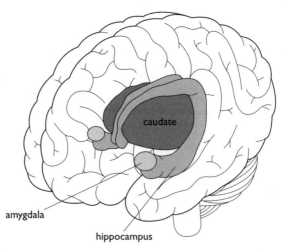

Figure 3 Three brain regions (among many) important for memory consolidation: hippocampus, caudate nucleus and amygdala.

The resolution of the 'place vs response' issue ultimately required information about the functions of different brain systems in learning and memory. We'll start with a brief discussion of two brain regions, the hippocampus and the caudate, that are now known to play roles in memory (see figure 3).

First the hippocampus. Studies of memory in the famous patient H.M. by the Canadian psychologist Brenda Milner provided the first evidence suggesting that the hippocampus is important for making new memories.[25] As a treatment for epilepsy, the anterior parts of H.M.'s hippocampus (as well as adjacent brain regions) were surgically removed on both sides of his brain. After the surgery, H.M. permanently lost the ability to retain explicit lasting memory of new experiences, but his ability to recall very recent experiences (i.e. primary memory) or well-learned remote experiences was relatively unimpaired. With the publication of these remarkable findings the hippocampus quickly became the main brain region of interest for studies of memory and has remained so for almost half a century.

In rats as well as primates (including, of course, human subjects), lesions of this brain region impair the storage or consolidation of new explicit knowledge such as facts and relationships between different kinds of new information, including the ability to make inferences based on acquired information and to remember the specific sequences of events.[26] I'll discuss hippocampal functioning in memory in more detail later.

Next the caudate, a brain region that is known to be important in regulating body movements. Dysfunction of this region is associated with disorders such as Parkinson's disease; and in rats, lesions here impair, relatively selectively, certain kinds of response learning. This issue is also discussed in more detail later on.

The mounting evidence that these two brain regions, the hippocampus and caudate, are involved in different kinds of learning suggested that there might be a more satisfactory resolution of the 'place vs response' issue studied and then abandoned decades ago. Maybe the rats in those studies learned *both* what response to make and *where* to go to find food – memories in conflict when tested by starting them from a different place in the testing room. Those early studies yielded an important but neglected clue. There was some evidence that response learning occurred when the rats were given extensive training in the T-maze before the test to determine whether they had learned to go to a place or make a turning response. Maybe that occurred because the extensive training increased the involvement of the caudate in the learning. Mark Packard and I obtained results that strongly suggest that this is what happened.[27]

The experiment we conducted was like the T-maze study described above. The rats were first trained in a T-maze with food as a reward. For the test the starting arm of the T was placed on the side of the room opposite to that used in the training (see figure 2). To examine the involvement of the hippocampus and caudate on memory for the training, we infused a small amount of the anaesthetic drug lidocaine into one of the two brain regions just before the animals were tested, in order to inactivate that specific brain region. Controls received infusions of a saline control solution. With but seven days of training on the T-maze (four trials per day) rats given saline infusions before

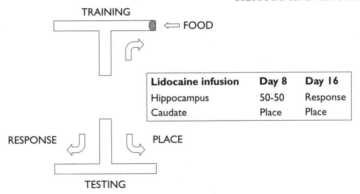

Lidocaine infused into the hippocampus or caudate before testing

Figure 4 The hippocampus and caudate are differentially involved in place and response learning at early and late stages of training. Rats were first trained to find food in one alley of a T maze. The maze was then rotated 180 degrees and the animals were tested for 'place' or 'response' learning. After eight days of training most of the animals went to the place, rather than making a right-turning response. After sixteen days of training, most animals made a turning response. Lidocaine infused into the hippocampus before the Day-8 test blocked place-going. Lidocaine infused into the caudate before the Day-16 test blocked the turning response seen in controls. From Packard and McGaugh, 1996.

the test went to the place where food had been found (see figure 4). In contrast, with fifteen days of training they made a turning response. Thus, with extensive training most of the animals shifted from going to 'place' to making a turning 'response'.

Very different results were found with rats given lidocaine infusions into the caudate or hippocampus before the tests. When they were tested after seven days, lidocaine infused into the caudate had no effect. That is, as with controls, they chose the food place. In contrast, rats given lidocaine infusions into the hippocampus behaved randomly. That memory of the place where reward was received was disrupted. These findings indicate that memory involving the hippocampus occurs earlier in training than that involving the striatum. With additional training the results were quite different. On the test given after fifteen days of training, rats given lidocaine infusions into the hippocampus behaved like saline controls: they made turning responses. However, rats given lidocaine infusions into the caudate did not make the well-trained turning response, but instead, went to the *place* where food had previously been found. Place memory very clearly remained intact throughout the extensive training and was revealed by inactivation of the caudate. Tolman was correct: there is more than one form of learning; but what he did not know is that different forms of learning coexist and that the expression of memory involves orchestration by different brain systems.

Most of us can certainly walk and chew gum at the same time. We can also listen to and learn and remember words or music (or words *and* music) while typing on a keyboard and sometimes do all of that while driving a car. We can do that because, like the rats' well-learned turning response in a maze, our over-learned responses also become somewhat automatic. When driving away from the University I sometimes end up in the driveway of my home when I intended to drive somewhere else (I suspect that you, too, have done something like that on occasion!); but although the general response I make – driving from the University to my home – is a well-practised one, the detailed sequences of motor responses made on each trip vary enormously, depending upon the traffic conditions, the weather and many other factors. Each detailed sequence of responses requires the integrative use of many kinds of memory. Also, like rats, we can go from one place to another by making unique sequences of responses based on our memory of the places and the possible routes between them as well as the responses required to use that information.

Brain systems – keeping track of memories and using them

Our brain has a tough job. It certainly does not use only ten per cent of its capacity, as has often been suggested. Our brain has continuously to take care of all of the ongoing vital housekeeping jobs such as seeing that we breathe, swallow, cough, sneeze, regulate body temperature, eat, maintain body posture and alternate sleep with wakefulness, just to name a few. In addition to these regulating and managing functions, we and the other animals have developed a great many specialized neural systems for sensing the world and for behaving in it. Different brain systems are responsible for detecting various kinds of sensory information and still others are responsible for enabling motor responses. At the same time that they are doing all of this, our brains have to insure that we acquire and retain all kinds of information, perhaps only briefly or perhaps for a lifetime, so that we can behave adaptively in response to changing events in our lives. Just as we have different systems for detecting sounds and sights, we also appear to have different brain systems enabling us to remember different kinds of information for different intervals of time.

As I discuss later, the processes enabling William James's primary, or short-term, memory differ from those underlying secondary, or long-term, memory; and, as we have just seen, even for long-term memory the brain systems involved in acquiring explicit memory of places differ from those involved in learning to make general responses such as turning responses in a maze. Yet another system enables the learning of more highly specific and restricted motor responses; but these are only parts of a much more complicated brain puzzle. Still other brain systems have other specialized jobs to do in making and retrieving memory of other kinds. For example, the eminent psychologist John Garcia discovered that we have a specialized and highly efficient brain system for learning that specific tastes and odours are associated with an upset stomach.[28] Hospital staff used to reward children with ice cream for undergoing radiation treatments for cancer. They stopped doing that when they discovered that the children stopped eating ice cream after receiving a few treatments. The children's brains concluded that the radiation-induced malaise was caused by the ice cream. Although it was the wrong conclusion in this instance, it is generally not a bad idea to conclude that if we have an upset stomach, it must have been caused by something that we ate – not something that we heard, saw or touched. As Garcia discovered, our brains draw that conclusion for us.

The past half-century of research has made it very clear that we do not have a single general system in our brains that is responsible for our learning and memory. What we learn depends on the kinds of information we encounter and the kinds of behaviour required. Although we know that different brain systems are involved in at least some different types of memory, there is much yet to be learned. We have to be cautious in discussing what we mean by 'involved in'; brain systems may serve many functions in learning and memory. They may be the place in the brain where certain kinds of memories are stored – that is, the locus of 'engrams'. They may be regions concerned with regulating the storage of memories. They may play special roles in retrieving memory. They may regulate the generation of learned responses. The only way to discover the role(s) is to do careful research designed to examine each possible role. Additionally, however, brain systems certainly must interact while performing all of these memory functions. Thus, memory research is very complicated detective work. Studies of animal as well as human memory are crucial in investigating brain functioning in memory; but, quite unlike the original reasons for studying animal learning discussed earlier in this chapter, animals are now studied because investigation of the neurobiological processes underlying memory in animals is essential for providing clues to memory systems and cellular processes in human brains. The extensive evidence that laboratory animals and humans use common brain systems and mechanisms is essential in the search for critical clues. As I discuss more extensively in the chapters that follow, many kinds of experiments using many kinds of research techniques are required to determine the functions and interactions among memory systems. Each new finding provides a clue suggesting new interim conclusions and new experiments to increase our understanding of how brain systems create, retain and retrieve memories appropriate for each occasion in our lives. Each clue is helping to solve the mystery of memory.

3 | The Short and the Long of It

'The stream of thought flows on; but most of its seg-
ments fall into the bottomless abyss of oblivion. Of
some, no memory survives the instant of their passage.
Of others, it is confined to a few moments, hours, or
days. Others, again, leave vestiges which are indestruct-
ible, and by means of which they may be recalled as
long as life endures. Can we explain these differences?'[1]

A graduate student in my laboratory was found lying uncon-
scious at the edge of the dry riverbed next to some rocks and his
broken bicycle. When he regained consciousness in the hospital
the next day, he did not know where he was or why he was
there. He had no memory of falling off his bicycle into the
riverbed. He did not even remember that he had ridden his
bicycle on the day of the accident or any other experiences of
that day: a brief segment of the record of his life was lost. The
memories of earlier experiences in his life, however, including
those of the day before the accident, were safe and sound. This
kind of selective memory loss is commonly seen after mild
head trauma, as well as with other conditions affecting brain
functioning. It is called 'retrograde amnesia', because the memories lost are those of events experienced before the trauma.
The older and stronger the memory, the less the loss. This
feature of memory loss, like the workers' union or personnel
policy 'Last hired, first fired', is known as 'Ribot's law', as it
was first discussed in the late nineteenth century by the French
psychologist Theodule Ribot.[2]

Ribot's law was also obeyed a couple of decades earlier when
I was on a skiing trip with some of my graduate students and
other laboratory colleagues. One of the students had one of

those 'highlight-film' falls and hit his head on the base of a tree. He got up, put his skis back on, said he was OK and then skied another couple of runs before telling us that he was not feeling well and needed to be taken home. It is particularly interesting that the head trauma did not impair his short-term (or primary) memory of the fall or events shortly after the fall. However, to this day he has no memory of that skiing trip – no memory of skiing before the fall, falling, or skiing after the fall. As with the graduate student who fell off his bicycle, this student also had (and still has) retrograde amnesia. In addition, he has 'antero-grade amnesia' – that is, even though he remained conscious after his fall, he lost memory of events, such as the ski runs after his fall, that occurred within a few hours *after* the acci-dent. Happily, the brain trauma and the lost memories were not critical for either of these students; both are now well-known neuroscientists.

In some cases the extent of the retrograde amnesia is clearly determined. In one such case a boxer in a four-round bout received a number of blows to his head but was not knocked out and did not appear to be dazed:

[Observers] remarked that he was fighting badly during his last round. He himself had no recollection of the last half of the third round nor of the last round…He could not judge the onset of his amnesia accurately but its end was sharply defined. It lasted between 15 and 20 minutes and during it he had shaken hands with his opponent, spoken to some of his friends and prepared himself for a shower.[3]

Making memories that last: memory consolidation

Although our early ancestors were no doubt the first to note that head trauma induced by accidents and aggressive encoun-ters can cause memory loss, systematic scientific study of amnesia began only in the last century. A study of two hundred patients who had had head injury reported that the patients generally had both retrograde and anterograde amnesia.[4] Moreover, the extent of the retrograde memory loss was greatest in those patients who had the most extensive memory loss for events occurring after the head trauma. It seems clear from anecdotal observations and clinical findings that long-term memories are initially highly fragile. In contrast, short-term memory is often unaffected by head trauma and other conditions that induce retrograde amnesia. These findings and others discussed below leave little doubt that James's primary (i.e. short-term) and secondary (i.e. long-term) memory are based on very different brain processes.

Why, though, are memories that are meant to be lasting so highly vulnerable to disruption immediately after learning and decreasingly vulnerable with the passage of time? A suggested explanation came from completely unrelated experimental findings. In 1900, two German psychologists, Georg Müller (a student of Ebbinghaus) and Alfons Pilzecker, found that memory for newly learned nonsense syllables was impaired by learning new ones shortly after the original learning.[5] Memory was not impaired, however, if some time was allowed to pass before the learning of the new syllables. To account for these findings they proposed that the memory traces of newly acquired information perseverate after learning and, over time, become consolidated. They suggested that the new learning occurring shortly after the original learning caused forgetting by disrupting the perseveration and, thus, the consolidation of the original learning. This was the first explicit theory of forgetting. It was almost immediately obvious to those who were familiar with clinical findings of head-trauma-induced memory loss that the consolidation hypothesis provided a possible explanation for retrograde amnesia.[6]

The consolidation hypothesis was largely ignored for almost half a century. Several developments unrelated to research on memory reignited interest in memory consolidation in the mid-1900s. Efforts to find treatments for severe psychiatric disorders, including depression and schizophrenia, played a seminal role. The stimulant drug camphor, administered in doses that induce convulsions, was first used for treating depression in the late eighteenth century. In the early 1930s there was a renewed interest in the use of convulsive drugs to treat psychiatric disorders, and injections of the synthetic drug metrazol or insulin replaced camphor as the convulsive treatment of choice. Two decades later I was a technician in a psychiatric hospital and witnessed patients, lying in rows of beds in an open ward, receiving injections of seizure-inducing doses of insulin (followed by infusions of glucose) as a treatment for their mental disorders. A major problem with such drug treatments, quite apart from the issue of whether they were safe and effective, was that the onset, degree and duration of the seizures were highly variable.

Two Italian psychiatrists, Cerletti and Bini, discovered a solution to that problem.[7] After observing that hogs in the Rome slaughterhouse were stunned, but not killed, by seizure-inducing electric current applied to their heads, they reasoned that it might be possible to use electrical stimulation to induce seizures in human patients. Luck was with them. The patient soon selected for their historic experiment was a man who was found wandering about the Rome train station in a confused state. After diagnosing their patient as having symptoms of schizophrenia they decided to administer electrical stimulation. Much to the relief of Cerletti and Bini (and the luck of the patient!) the electroshock stimulation induced a convulsion and did not kill the patient. Electroconvulsive shock (ECS), now termed electroconvulsive therapy (ECT) when used with human patients, was soon widely accepted as a treatment for mental disorders and is still used as an effective treatment for some types of severe depression not alleviated by antidepressant drugs. I met Cerletti when I was doing postdoctoral research in Rome but, unfortunately, did not take advantage of the occasion to ask him about his historic 'experiment'. I say 'unfortunately' because, at the time, I was using ECS treatments to study memory consolidation in rats and I missed the opportunity to discuss with him his memory of that pioneering event that influenced my own research and continues to influence research on memory today.

What is the connection between ECT, or ECS, and memory? Soon after ECT was adopted as a treatment for mental disorders it was noted that patients given ECT treatments had impaired memory, especially for events occurring shortly before or after each treatment – that is, it seemed that the patients had both retrograde and anterograde amnesia. These clinical findings suggested that it might be possible to use electroshock stimulation as an experimental technique to study memory consolidation. That idea was examined in a classic experiment by Carl Duncan published in 1949.[8] Rats in that study were trained, on a number of days, to avoid a footshock by moving from one compartment in an apparatus to another at the onset of a signal. Rats in different groups received ECS treatments at one of several delay intervals after the daily training trial. Those given an ECS treatment within a few seconds after training showed no evidence of memory of the training experience. In contrast, the performance of rats given the ECS treatment at intervals of one hour or longer after training was unimpaired. The finding that the post-training treatment effect on memory was time-dependent provided strong experimental support for the long-neglected memory consolidation hypothesis.

Duncan's study immediately stimulated a cascade of laboratory experiments investigating the effects of ECS on memory. The aim of much of the early research was to determine the time required for memory consolidation or, as it was termed, the consolidation gradient. However, the search for 'the' memory consolidation gradient proved to be elusive and, ultimately, ill-advised. The length of the gradient turned out to depend upon the particular conditions used in any experiment. The gradients varied from seconds to days, depending on many variables, including the learning task, type of training, strain of rats and, especially, the specific post-training treatment used to induce the retrograde amnesia.[9] The retrograde amnesia found in such

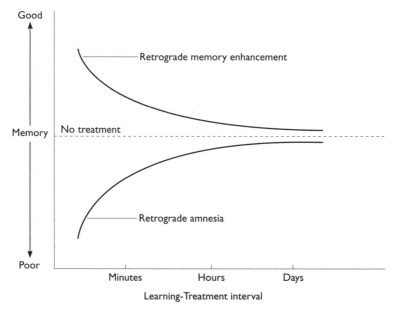

Figure 5 Effects, on memory consolidation, of treatments given at different times after learning. Upper curve: retrograde enhancement of memory. Lower curve: retrograde amnesia.

studies is represented in the lower part of figure 5. The major contribution of Duncan's study was the finding that it is possible to study memory consolidation experimentally. It was, and is, no longer necessary to rely solely on clinical and anecdotal reports.

The dual-trace hypothesis: fragile to stable memories?

The highly influential book *Organization of Behavior* by the Canadian psychologist D. O. Hebb (1949)[10] also helped to rekindle interest in memory consolidation. By coincidence, Hebb's book was published in the same year as Duncan's classic study. In his book Hebb proposed what he called a 'dual-trace' hypothesis of memory:

To the extent that anatomical and physiological observations establish the possibility of reverberatory after-effects of a sensory event, it is established that such a process would be the physiological basis of a transient 'memory' of the stimulus. To account for...permanence, some structural change seems necessary, but a structural growth presumably would require an appreciable time. The conception of a transient, unstable reverberatory trace is therefore useful, if it is possible to suppose that some more permanent structural change reinforces it.[11]

The dual-trace hypothesis is, quite obviously, remarkably similar to Müller and Pilzecker's long-neglected perseveration–consolidation hypothesis. Thus, it is of interest that Hebb did not discuss or even cite that hypothesis. Both hypotheses propose that long-term memory is formed by stabilizing the memory trace established immediately after an experience – that is, over time the initially fragile trace becomes a durable trace. Short-term memory simply becomes long-lasting. For both hypotheses the difference between short- and long-term memory is simply the strength of the memory trace. Thus, it would be more accurate to consider the consolidation and dual-trace hypotheses as *single-trace* hypotheses. We now have good reason to believe that these hypotheses, however influential, are wrong – or, more conservatively, as discussed below, there is compelling evidence that recent and remote memory are based on different processes, not the same process differing only in durability. However, there is also extensive evidence that the hypotheses were partly correct: lasting memories are not created instantly; they consolidate over time.

Birds do it, bees do it – even molluscs, fish and fleas do it

Many studies using many kinds of post-training treatment affecting brain functioning have contributed greatly to our understanding of brain processes underlying the creation of lasting memories. In pioneering studies using goldfish, Bernard Agranoff found that, like ECS, protein synthesis inhibitors injected after training produce retrograde amnesia.[12] In other experiments he

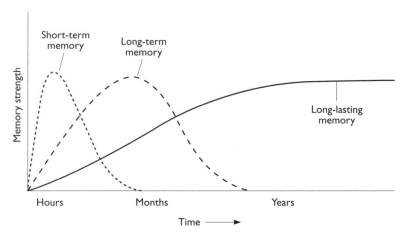

Figure 6 Stages of memory formation. Memory consolidation is time-dependent; however, different stages of memory are not sequentially linked but are based on independent processes operating in parallel. Modified from McGaugh, 1966; McGaugh, 2000.

administered protein synthesis inhibitors immediately *before* the fish were trained. The remarkable finding was that the fish learned the task completely normally but forgot it within a few hours – that is, the protein synthesis inhibitors blocked memory consolidation but did not influence short-term memory. There is now extensive evidence that short-term memory is spared by many kinds of treatments (including ECT) that block memory consolidation. Additionally, and equally importantly, the Argentinian/Brazilian neuroscientist Ivan Izquierdo found that many drug treatments can block short-term memory without blocking memory consolidation.[13] Contrary to Hebb's hypothesis, long-term memory does not require short-term memory. Such findings suggest, as is shown in figure 6, that parallel and possibly independent stages of memory, each with a different life span, are created by our experiences.

All of this evidence from clinical and experimental studies strongly indicates that the brain handles recent and remote memory in different ways; but why does it do that? We obviously need to have memory that is created rapidly. Reacting to an ever and rapidly changing environment requires that. How could we converse, read, or even walk, if all memory developed slowly after each experience? Most current building codes, for example, require that the heights of all steps in a staircase be equal. After taking a couple of steps, up or down, we implicitly remember the heights of the steps and assume that the others will be the same. If they are not the same, we are very likely to trip and fall. Lack of this kind of rapidly created implicit memory would be bad for us and for insurance companies, but perhaps good for lawyers. It would be of little value to us if we remembered the heights of the steps only after a delay of many hours, when the memory becomes consolidated. Or, imagine having a conversation in which interchanges can occur only at intervals of an hour or so. Having a quickly created memory appears to be a very good idea. Of course, responding only after an interval of a couple of hours can be very useful (and well-advised) if there are things to mull over carefully before responding; but mulling over requires short-term memory.

The hypothesis that lasting memory consolidates slowly over time is supported primarily by clinical and experimental evidence that the formation of long-term memory is influenced by treatments and disorders affecting brain functioning; but there are also other kinds of evidence indicating more directly that the memories consolidate over time after learning. Avi Karni and Dov Sagi[14] in Israel reported that the performance of human subjects trained in a visual skill did not improve until eight hours after the training was completed and that improvement was even greater the following day. Furthermore, the skill was retained for several years. Studies using human brain imaging to study changes in neural activity induced by learning have also reported that the changes continue to develop for hours after learning. In an innovative study using functional imagining of the brain by PET (positron emission tomography), Reza Shadmehr and Henry Holcomb[15] examined brain activity in several brain regions shortly after human subjects were trained in a motor learning task requiring arm and hand movements. They found that while subjects' performance remained stable for several hours after completion of the training, their brain activity did not; different regions of the brain were predominantly active at different times over a period of several hours after the training. The activity shifted from the prefrontal cortex to two areas known to be involved in controlling movements, the motor cortex and cerebellar cortex. Consolidation of the motor skill appeared to involve activation of different neural systems that increased the stability of the brain processes underlying the skill.

There is also evidence that learning-induced changes in the activity of neurons in the cerebral cortex continue to increase for many days after the training. In an extensive series of electrophysiological studies using rats with electrodes implanted in the auditory cortex,[16] Norman Weinberger reported that, after a tone of specific frequency was paired a few times with footshock, neurons in the rats' auditory cortex responded *more* to that specific tone and *less* to other tones of other frequencies. Even more interestingly, the selectivity of the neurons' response to the specific tone used in training continued to increase for several days after the training was terminated. These findings suggest that the memory of the tone's increased significance continued to consolidate long after the training was finished.[17]

It is not intuitively obvious why our lasting memories consolidate slowly. Certainly one can wonder why we have a form of memory that we have to rely on for remembering for many hours, days or a lifetime, that is so susceptible to disruption shortly after it is initiated. Perhaps the brain system that consolidates long-term memory over time was a late development in vertebrate evolution. Moreover, maybe we consolidate memories slowly because our mammalian brains are large and enormously complex. We can readily reject these ideas. All species of animals studied to date have both short- and long-term memory; and all are susceptible to retrograde amnesia. Birds, bees, and molluscs, as well as fish and rats (as noted above), like us, make long-term memory slowly.[18] Consolidation of memory clearly emerged early in evolution and was conserved.

Although there seems to be no compelling reason to conclude that a biological system such as our brain could not quickly make a lasting memory, the fact is that animal brains do not. Thus, memory consolidation must serve some very important adaptive function or functions. As I discuss extensively in a later chapter, there is considerable evidence suggesting that the slow consolidation is adaptive because it enables neurobiological processes occurring shortly after learning to influence the strength of memory for experiences. The extensive evidence, discussed in subsequent chapters, that memory can be *enhanced*, as well as impaired, by treatments administered shortly after training provides intriguing support for this hypothesis. So we will subsequently return to that important issue.

Passing fancies that in time may go

We are continuously learning new information moment by moment and integrating it with traces of recent and long-past experiences. We remember the last few words just read and the last few words just spoken. We can distinguish each of these from words read and spoken yesterday. Yet yesterday, today and even thoughts about tomorrow can be brought together and can mingle together, forming new memories: memory traces interact and accumulate in our brains. Imagine, if you can, what your life would be like if you were to lose, at this very moment, the ability to consolidate traces of new experiences in long-term memory. This critical ability is, in fact, lost by patients with brain damage induced by many kinds of diseases and disorders. In degenerative diseases such as Alzheimer's the loss may occur gradually over many years. With other conditions, such as brain injury, hypoxia or encephalitis, the onset of the impaired memory may be sudden. Whether slow or sudden in onset, the consequence is catastrophic:

Such patients therefore who no longer fix the present live constantly in a past which preceded the onset of their illness. Their disengagement from the present is, however, far from complete. Some are conscious of the disorder, like [one patient], who said: 'When I watch closely I know, but I soon forget. My brain feels like a sieve, I forget everything. Even in my tiny room, I keep losing things. It all fades away.'[19]

H.M, the patient discussed briefly in the preceding chapter, is by far the most well-studied amnesic patient.[20] Because the findings of studies of his memory have so profoundly influenced thinking and research on memory consolidation and other aspects of memory for so many decades, I need to provide a few more facts concerning his history. His case is yet another example of how an attempt to deal with a problem unrelated to memory has provided deep insights into memory. H.M.'s problem began with the onset of minor seizures when he was six years old, and became more severe at age sixteen, when he began to have major seizures. At the age of twenty-seven, both the frequency and severity of the seizures had greatly increased and could not be controlled by medication. It was known that surgical removal of the brain regions in which the seizures originated could often alleviate or reduce them. Thus, in an effort to treat the seizure disorder, brain surgery was performed and the medial parts of both temporal lobes of his brain were excised. Within a few days after the surgery it became obvious that his memory was severely impaired; but, very interestingly, as discussed below, it was not *completely* impaired.

> He could no longer recognize the hospital staff...he did not remember and could not relearn the way to the bathroom, and he seemed to retain nothing of the day-to-day happenings in the hospital. His early memories were seemingly vivid and intact, his speech was normal, and his social behaviour and emotional responses were entirely appropriate. ...[he] will do the the same jigsaw puzzles day after day without showing any practice effect, and read the same magazines over and over again without finding their contents familiar.
>
> Even such profound amnesias as this are, however, compatible

with a normal attention span...On one occasion he was asked to remember the number '584' and was then allowed to sit quietly with no interruption for 15 minutes, at which point he was able to recall the number...When asked how he had been able to do this he replied, 'It's easy you just remember 8. You see, 5, 8, and 4 add to 17. You remember 8; subtract it from 17 and it leaves 9. Divide 9 in half and you get 5 and 4, and there you are, 584. Easy.'...[he] was unable, a minute or so later to remember the number '584'...in fact, he did not know that he had been given a number to remember. Between tests he would suddenly look up and say...'Right now, I'm wondering. Have I said or done anything amiss? You see, at this moment everything looks clear to me, but what happened just before? That's what worries me. It's like waking up from a dream; I just don't remember.'[21]

H.M.'s explicit memory for recent experiences quickly faded away. When asked to say whether two sounds or lights presented in sequence were the same or different, he made few errors when twenty seconds elapsed between the stimuli and, unlike normal subjects, performed poorly with a sixty-second delay. H.M.'s explicit memory, unlike that of normal human subjects, did not benefit from repetition; for him, practice did not make perfect. He could, for a short period of time, remember a maximum of six numbers and could not learn a series of numbers longer than six even if the series was repeated many times.

Memory without remembering

Suzanne Corkin's study of H.M.'s memory over the past several decades clearly indicates, however, that H.M. has been able to learn some kinds of information.[22] He was able to learn several types of 'implicit' perceptual memory tasks as well as some specific, explicit information. Five years after his operation he moved to a different house and lived there until 1974. When tested in 1966 and again in 1977, three years after moving from that house, he was able to remember the street address as well as the layout of the rooms in that house, which he moved to *after* his brain surgery. Thus, although H.M. lacked the ability to acquire lasting memory of specific events (episodic memory), his capacity to learn at least some general information was spared.

Another patient, E.P., studied by Edmond Teng and Larry Squire,[23] has extensive bilateral damage of his hippocampus and adjacent temporal lobe regions. This patient is so amnesic that he is unable to recognize those who have tested him over forty times during the course of a year. Additionally, he has no knowledge of the neighbourhood in which he currently lives but moved to after the onset of his amnesia. In contrast, E.P.'s memory of how to get around in a town where he lived earlier in his life but which he moved away from over fifty years previously is unimpaired. Clearly, the brain damage that impairs his ability to acquire new information did not destroy spatial information acquired fifty years earlier. Additionally, these findings, like those of the study of H.M.'s memory of the floor plan of the house he had lived in after his surgery, very clearly indicate that an intact hippocampal system is not required for the retrieval of spatial information.

As noted above, despite his inability to learn new explicit information, H.M. was able to learn and remember some implicit information. He was taught, on three successive days, to trace a line within a star-shaped pattern while viewing his hand and the pattern in a mirror. He improved each day, beginning at the level achieved at the end of the preceding day, even though from day to day he did not remember that he had previously performed the task, and retained the skill for at least a year. Subsequent studies of amnesic patients have provided extensive evidence that memory for various kinds of implicit information is often unimpaired. In an early classic study, for example, the British psychologists Elizabeth Warrington and Lawrence Weiskrantz[24] showed amnesic patients a series of five pictures of each of several common objects, such as an aeroplane, or a word, on three successive days. The initial figures were only fragments and thus could not be identified by either normal subjects or amnesic patients. Each successive picture was more complete and the fifth was readily identifiable. After the amnesic patients were given repeated trials administered on three days of testing, they were able to identify the objects or words when shown the highly fragmented incomplete figures. These amnesic patients, like H.M., displayed memory without remembering. Larry Squire and his colleagues[25] have reported that amnesic patients can have an intact 'implicit' learning ability even though they lack explicit memory of the tasks they have learned or that they have learned them. They can, for example, learn and retain the skill of reading words presented in mirror image. Also, when shown words such as 'absent' or 'income' they will subsequently complete the words correctly when presented with 'abs___' or 'in___', when asked to form the first word that comes to mind, even though they cannot remember having seen the words.

Studies of amnesic patients clearly support William James's distinction between short- and long-term memory. Short-term memory can be, and usually is, relatively intact in amnesic patients. Additionally, such studies reveal that damage to medial temporal lobe structures, including the hippocampus and adjacent regions of the cerebral cortex, impairs the consolidation of explicit memory. However, they also reveal that some forms of implicit memory are spared, even in seriously amnesic patients. Thus, other brain regions appear to be responsible for mediating the consolidation of forms of implicit learning, including some perceptual-cognitive information and motor skills. These pioneering studies of memory in amnesic patients were seminal in stimulating research investigating the roles of different brain systems in mediating different forms of memory. They also raise interesting important questions. What is the function of such implicit memory – remembering without explicit remembering? It seems likely that such learning is critical – and perhaps even sufficient – for acquiring many kinds of skills. Certainly that must be true for motor skill learning, simply because the learning consists *of* the motor skill. Explicit remembering of the skill and the learning of it may play no essential role in performance of the skill. Do we, like amnesic patients, all have a private world of learning and memory that is not accessible to conscious experience? It appears that we do. Our explicit memory may mislead us as we provide explanations of our own behaviour. The amnesic patient who has seen the word 'HOTEL' may say, as an explanation of why he or she responded with the letters 'HO' when presented with '___TEL' a few hours later, 'I'm just good at word games.' Were we to be asked the same question, we would probably say that we responded with 'HO' because we *remember* having seen the word 'HOTEL' a few hours previously. Certainly such a response of an amnesic patient would be creative but wrong. Would our response be any *less* creative and wrong? Maybe not.

Long ago and far away

As discussed above, and as I will discuss more extensively later in the book, most studies of consolidation focus on processes occurring over a period of several hours or days after learning. However, the findings of clinical studies suggest that memory consolidation may continue for years. Brain damage resulting from such conditions as brain injury, encephalitis, a stroke or reduction in blood or oxygen supply to the brain can sometimes induce retrograde amnesia for events occurring years, or even decades, earlier. The amnesic patient E.P. discussed above had great difficulty remembering experiences that occurred in the forty years prior to the onset of his amnesia. Another patient who had had severe brain injury, '...on returning home was quite unable to recall that her house had been redecorated about six months before her accident and expressed much surprise at its spick-and-span appearance...recollection of the weeks or months preceding a severe head injury [is] often found to be vague and somewhat sketchy.'[26]

A number of years ago a neuroscientist friend of mine told me this story about his mother. He was working in his laboratory with a visiting colleague from Hungary when he received a telephone message that his mother had had a severe stroke and been taken to a hospital, where she had been placed in intensive care. The hospital staff were extremely concerned because, although his mother was conscious, she was 'babbling' incoherently. My friend and his visiting colleague rushed to the hospital. Within a few minutes the visiting colleague began to tell the nurses what my friend's mother had been trying, without success, to tell them for the previous couple of hours. He was able to do this because she was speaking Hungarian. My friend's mother had immigrated to the United States when she was a teenager and had spoken only English for decades. After she had the stroke she was no longer able to speak English and reverted to her first language, which was completely preserved. Unfortunately, I did not learn whether her retrograde amnesia extended more generally, to other things she had learned during the decades before her stroke, or was restricted selectively to loss of the ability to speak English.

The initial findings that led to the proposal of the perseveration-consolidation hypothesis were based on studies of retention of material learned only a few minutes prior to the retention test. Experimental studies of retrograde amnesia have generally reported gradients of retrograde amnesia extending only for a few hours or days. Those findings suggest that memory consolidation is largely completed within hours, or perhaps days at the most. How, then, are the findings of clinical studies of retrograde amnesia for explicit memory extending over decades to be interpreted?[27] Do the memory consolidation processes activated by an experience continue throughout our lifetimes? Are the conditions that induce very long gradients more effective in producing amnesia simply because they are more effective in disrupting critical brain processes? It seems highly unlikely (though perhaps not impossible) that the specific neural processes initiated by each of our experiences last and consolidate slowly over our lifetimes. If consolidation worked that way, why would we have any lasting memories? Retrograde amnesia would be the rule rather than the exception. It also seems highly unlikely that the experimental treatments used in studies of retrograde amnesia are in all cases less disruptive of brain processes than are naturally occurring injuries and diseases that induce long gradients of retrograde amnesia. Some other explanation(s) for decades-long gradients seem required.

A clue provided by studies of H.M. and other amnesic patients suggests that the hippocampus and related brain regions in the medial temporal cortex may be critically important in enabling long-term consolidation of explicit memory in the cerebral cortex. It might be that the explicit information is first held in the hippocampus and then transferred to the cortex. Alternatively, the hippocampus may regulate the organization of neural memory traces in cortical regions. According to either of these views, the cortex gradually, over time, becomes independent of the organizational influences provided by the hippocampal system.[28] These explanations of long gradients of retrograde amnesia suggest that the hippocampal system has very long-lasting regulating influences on the development and integration of memory traces in the cortex. These very long-term effects are represented in the curve on the far right in figure 6. This later stage of memory consolidation involving hippocampal system–cortical interactions builds on an earlier stage of memory consolidation occurring within hours or days after learning. This view is based on evidence that the hippocampal system is involved in the consolidation of explicit (episodic) information; but, as discussed above, we know that other forms of memory do not require the hippocampal system. Thus, any evidence of very long-term gradients of retrograde amnesia for perceptual-motor skills and other forms of implicit learning would require some other explanation. Unfortunately, at present little is known about retrograde amnesia for skills and other forms of implicit knowledge.

Most reports of very long-term retrograde amnesia are based on

studies of memory in patients with brain damage; but experimental studies have also contributed some important findings. Larry Squire and his colleagues found that patients given a
series of ECT treatments had retrograde amnesia for information
acquired during the most recent two or three years prior to the
treatments.[29] In animals, lesions of the hippocampus can produce
retrograde amnesia for training that occurred several weeks or
months before the lesions were induced. In one study examining
this issue,[30] Jeansok Kim and Michael Fanselow gave rats a series
of footshocks in an apparatus and studied their memory by assess-
ing the animals' 'freezing' behaviour thirty-five days later when
they were replaced in the apparatus where they had received the
footshocks. In animals in different groups, hippocampal lesions
were induced one, seven, fourteen or twenty-eight days after the
training. The retention performance of animals given the lesions
twenty-eight days after training was like that of normal, non-
lesioned rats. In contrast, rats given hippocampal lesions one day
after training showed no evidence of memory of the training and
the performance of those given lesions seven or fourteen days
after training, although better than the one-day group, was worse
than that of the twenty-eight-day group. This evidence of retrograde amnesia extending over intervals of weeks supports the
hypothesis that the hippocampus is involved in the consolidation
of memory for this kind of training but that the involvement is
time-limited. After a month the hippocampus is no longer
required either for the storage or for the retrieval of the information. Thus, the findings are similar to those found with human
patients, although there is a great difference in the time scale:
weeks vs years. The findings are more similar, of course, if we
consider the length of the gradient of retrograde amnesia in relation to the life spans of the animal and human subjects. This
comparison assumes that memory processes in animals are scaled
to the animals' life spans. This is an intriguing hypothesis that
has not, as yet, been systematically considered.

Encoding episodic events: brain activity and lasting memory

In amnesic patients the link between short-term and long-term explicit memory is missing. New experiences do not leave lasting traces. The hippocampal complex in the medial temporal lobe appears to be the missing link. As discussed above, studies of amnesic patients and animals with lesions of the hippocampal complex strongly suggest that this brain region plays a critical time-limited role in consolidating lasting explicit memory. As discussed in a subsequent chapter, this conclusion is also supported by findings that certain drugs injected into this brain region can enhance long-term explicit memory.

For at least decades, and probably much longer than that, scientists have tried to imagine what the workings of the brain might look like when memories are created. If only we could, by some magic, peer though the skull and see the actions of different brain regions and the interactions between them that construct memories from our experiences. Well, some modern non-invasive brain imaging techniques, including PET and fMRI (functional magnetic resonance imaging), are beginning to allow us to do just that. But while these allow the creation of functional images of brain activity, it is quite another matter, and a much more complicated one, to use the images to decipher what the brain images tell us about the functioning of specific brain regions in memory. Peering alone won't do the job. Staring at the brain or images of brain activity won't tell anyone how our brains create memory. The peering has to be an interrogation – that is, brain activity is another kind of performance measure, albeit a very special and important kind of performance, which needs to be *critically* linked, by experimental evidence, to memory.

The findings of several brain-imaging studies support the conclusions based on lesion studies.[31] Long-term memory for words and photographs varies directly with the activity of a specific region of the medial temporal lobe, the parahippocampal gyrus, during the encoding of the material. In one of the studies, for example, Michael Alkire and his colleagues[32] recorded the subjects' brain activity, using PET, as the subjects listened passively to sequences of emotionally neutral, unrelated words. Memory for the words was tested the following day. Activity of the parahippocampal gyrus assessed during the encoding (i.e. passive listening) correlated highly (+0.91) with the number of words subsequently recalled – that is, the amount of brain activity during the learning predicted the memory tested the next day.[33]

These brain-imaging techniques currently do not allow us to find out whether, as the lesion studies suggest, the hippocampal complex remains active for very long periods of time after encoding of specific information. From a practical perspective it is difficult to see how such information would be obtained, because under ordinary circumstances human subjects continually encode and consolidate new information. Sorting the newer memory-induced brain activity from the older memory activity is a daunting task, at best. The research of Norman Weinberger, discussed above, revealed that learning-induced changes in the responsiveness of neurons in specific regions of the auditory cortex continued for many days after training and that the neurons continued to increase their selectivity in responding to a specific, significant tone (see references 16, 17). The finding that the continuing (consolidating) neural changes were monitored by recording electrophysiological responses from implanted electrodes suggests that brain-imaging techniques might be able to monitor long-lasting learning-induced neuronal activity underlying the consolidation of specific memories. In the only study, to date, that has used brain imaging to investigate this issue, Frank Haist and his colleagues[34] reported evidence, from fMRI imaging, suggesting that the hippocampus may participate in consolidation processes for a few years but that the adjacent entorhinal cortex participates for decades. However, for the present, the hypothesis that the hippocampal complex is involved in memory consolidation for an extensive period of time relies primarily on clinical and experimental studies of the effects of damage and disorders affecting the functioning of the hippocampal complex.

Interestingly, Eleanor Maguire and her colleagues in London[35] reported findings suggesting that extensive use of the hippocampus may alter its structure. Using MRI imaging, they examined the sizes of the hippocampus of experienced London taxi drivers, who are required to know the map of London in detail. The posterior hippocampal region of taxi drivers was slightly larger than that of comparable control subjects who did not have extensive navigational experience. In contrast, the anterior hippocampal region was larger in the control subjects. Further, the volumes of the taxi drivers' anterior and posterior hippocampal regions tended to vary (modestly) with the months of taxi driving experience (correlations of –0.60 and +0.50, respectively). In a study using fMRI to assess brain activation, Maguire and her colleagues also found that the right hippocampus of taxi drivers was activated when they were asked to recall complex routes on London streets. Although these findings seem to suggest that a large and functionally activated posterior hippocampus (and a smaller anterior hippocampus) may be required for successful taxi driving, these findings by themselves don't allow that conclusion. The findings of Teng and Squire (see reference 23), that patient E.P, who had extensive bilateral hippocampal damage, had no difficulty remembering the street layout of a town where he had lived fifty years before the occurrence of the hippocampal damage, indicate that an intact hippocampus is not required for recalling well-learned spatial information. Thus, although the findings of animal as well as human studies leave little doubt that the hippocampus is involved in acquiring relational information, there is little evidence suggesting that the hippocampus is the *locus* of the changes underlying long-term memory. Although using the hippocampus may alter its structure, it is not yet clear that such anatomical alteration results in better functioning; the change in size may simply reflect an increased use in consolidating new relational information stored elsewhere in the brain. But that conclusion, alone, would be extremely important.

Memory: short and long reprise

William James was correct: primary and secondary memory are
different forms of memory; they are based on different brain
processes. For most of us, as well as amnesic patients, recently
acquired memories often simply fade away. Detailed records of
daily experiences are kept mostly in diaries or perhaps recorded
in the latest model hand-held computers; but we do, quite obviously, have lasting memories. Those memories are not made
instantly but, as discussed above, are consolidated slowly over
time. Our long-term memories vary in detail and in strength.
The chapters that follow examine the conditions and brain
processes responsible for regulating the creation of strong, long-
lasting memories.

4 | Coaxing Consolidation: Making Memories Linger

Several years ago, an acquaintance asked me for the name of a drug that she could give to her child to improve the child's learning and memory. I wondered why she would want to give her child such a drug, as the child did not have any obvious disorder of learning or memory. However, the reason seemed clear enough: as drugs are routinely and extensively used to relieve pain, maintain alertness and decrease anxiety and depression, why not use one to improve learning and memory and thus aid a child's education – better memory through chemistry?

There are, as yet, no drugs suitable for enhancing children's learning and memory. Moreover, there are no drugs suitable for enhancing adults' memory – except for some used in the treatment of Alzheimer's disease. However, there is little doubt that there is considerable interest in discovering drugs that will improve learning and memory in normal children and adults. In the years since I was asked that question, I have asked many friends and neighbours whether they would take a memory-enhancing drug and/or give it to their children if there were one known to be safe and effective. Generally (with but rare exceptions) the answer has been a rather quick, 'Yes.' You might wonder, with good cause, why I bothered to ask, when so many products available today have names that suggest that they are memory boosters. The problem is that although sales of these products provide good evidence of very strong interest in improving customers' learning and memory, there is very little credible evidence that any of the enticing products currently offered can do so. Moreover, some of the products may impair memory, or have other potentially harmful effects, when taken with other commonly used drugs.

There are, as I noted above, several drugs approved for the treatment of memory disorders such as Alzheimer's disease; but these drugs are not yet highly effective and are most certainly not ones that you would recommend to neighbours and acquaintances – or their children – who do not have memory disorders. Pharmaceutical and biotech companies are currently investing many millions of dollars per year in attempts to develop new memory-enhancing drugs that will be effective in treating disordered and/or declining memory. As such drugs are developed, and found to be safe as well as effective and to have acceptable side effects, they will no doubt be of interest to (that is, sought by) many who simply want to improve their memory. Whether such drugs, when developed, should be used by those of us who *do not* have memory disorders is a highly complex issue with many social implications. Imagine, for example, putting memory-boosting pills in a child's lunch box, next to the peanut-butter sandwich and apple juice. If this should eventually happen, let's hope that the pills are very safe, very cheap and are available to all; but if they are available to *all*, why bother? Also, before reaching for the pills we should consider the critically important question of whether it is a good idea to make strong memories of *all* of our experiences. Do we really need to remember what we had for lunch two weeks ago last Thursday? Probably not; we do not need to have stronger memories of all of our experiences. Moreover, as I discuss in a later chapter, total recall may not be a good thing to have: it might well create cognitive chaos. However, if something important happened at that lunch two weeks ago last Thursday, then it is probably worth remembering. Perhaps a winning lottery ticket was discovered. Or maybe there was an angry interchange or a marriage proposal, or perhaps both, during the lunch. Or maybe the food was exceptionally good or bad. All of these possibilities would clearly be worth remembering, as they have important consequences for future actions. Thus, what we need is *selectively* enhanced memories of our *significant* experiences. Fortunately, as is discussed in the next chapter, nature figured out a way to enable our brains to achieve this for us.

As discussed in the previous chapter, many drugs disrupt the formation of long-term memory. Can drugs also improve learning and memory? This question has been asked in many studies using laboratory animals, mostly rats and mice. The answer is yes but, as we will see, a somewhat complex yes. The aim of most research investigating drug effects on learning and memory is only remotely or indirectly concerned with finding drugs to enhance human memory. Rather, the major purpose of most such research is to use drugs as investigative tools, together with many other techniques, to discover the neural mechanisms underlying learning and memory. Studies of drug effects on learning and memory have provided critical clues to the mechanisms that cause significant experiences to leave lasting memories. To consider how such research has provided important insights into the neural systems involved in creating long-term memory, we first need to consider a little historical background, some critical, conceptual and methodological issues, and a few experimental findings.

Stimulating learning

The first experiment investigating drug enhancement of learning was published in 1917 by the psychologist Karl Lashley.[1] Rats were trained in a maze with several alleys and, at the end of each trial, they found food in the final, correct alley. A few minutes before each daily training session, the rats were injected with either a solution of saline or a solution of saline containing the stimulant drug strychnine. The specific question asked by Lashley's experiment was whether low, sub-convulsive doses of this stimulant drug would improve the rate at which the animals learned the maze. The answer was yes: rats given strychnine before each training session were better at learning the maze than were rats given only the saline injections. They made fewer errors (entrances of incorrect alleys) on each training session and required fewer training trials to learn the correct maze path.

At that time, low doses of strychnine were commonly found in many over-the-counter patent medicines, or 'tonics'; but it is essential to know that strychnine was, and is, used as rat poison. In very low doses it is a central nervous system stimulant and in higher doses induces convulsions and death. Moreover, it is essential to note that most of the drugs used in experimental studies of memory enhancement discussed later cannot, or should not, be taken by any human subjects. The drugs are useful only for providing insights into memory mechanisms.

When we were graduate students at the University of California, Berkeley in the mid-1950s, Lewis Petrinovich and I discovered Lashley's paper while doing library research for a graduate seminar on brain chemistry and behaviour. This paper was particularly interesting to us because it was the only study, to our knowledge, reporting that a drug enhanced learning. To determine whether these results could be replicated, we repeated the experiment and were very pleased to obtain similar results.[2] The findings of these two experiments *seemed* quite clear: a low dose of a drug that stimulated the brain enhanced learning and memory; but is that really what the findings indicated? No, not necessarily. We, like Lashley, found only that the maze-*performance* of animals given the drug before training was better than that of the saline controls. It was an *inference* that the improved performance might have been due to improved learning and memory. The drug might simply have improved the rats' performance in the maze for some other reason or reasons.

The distinction between *learning* and *performance* (first emphasized by Edward Tolman[3]) is critical for understanding and interpreting such experimental findings. The drug might have enhanced maze performance by improving sensory systems (e.g. vision, smell, touch, etc.), alertness, attention, motor ability, or any of a large number of other processes that could influence rats' maze performance. Of course, if one is only interested in having rats that perform better in a maze, then there is no need to be concerned about the basis or bases of the improvement: animal trainers are not known for their interests in the learning/performance distinction; but if one is interested, as we were, in knowing whether the drug enhanced learning and memory, the experimental findings were only suggestive; there remained too many alternative interpretations. In the intervening years a great many studies have reported additional evidence that drugs administered to animals before training can enhance learning performance. Unfortunately, additional evidence of that kind is neither interesting nor useful, as it does not provide any critical insights into the basis or bases of the enhanced performance.

Consolidating clues

How can drug enhancement of memory be investigated without having to deal with the complications of the learning/performance problem? Findings discussed in chapter 3 revealed that electroconvulsive shock treatments administered within an hour or so after training produce retrograde amnesia, supporting the idea that learning-activated neural activity continuing for some time after training consolidates lasting memory. These results thus suggested a way of investigating drug enhancement of memory without having to worry about performance effects. If neural processes continuing after training are critical for long-term memory consolidation, then, I reasoned, it might be possible to enhance memory consolidation by administering stimulant drugs shortly *after* training. The learning/performance problem would thus be avoided because the animals would not be under the direct influence of the drugs during either the training or the subsequent testing for memory of the training. The drugs would influence brain activity *after* the training session, while the animals were resting quietly in their home cages, and would be eliminated (metabolized and excreted) within a few hours, well before the retention test the following day.

With the idea that a stimulant drug might selectively enhance the consolidation of memory for recent experiences freshly in mind, I rushed, with great enthusiasm, to the office of one of my graduate research advisors and told him about my idea. A rough and highly edited translation of his response and advice is that it was a bad idea and that I should forget about it. It was a short discussion. So I waited until he departed for a sabbatical leave in Europe before I conducted the first experiment to investigate the effects on long-term memory of administering a stimulant drug to rats immediately *after* training. In this experiment, some rats received injections of a saline control solution and others received one of several doses of the strychnine immediately after each daily training trial in the same alley maze as Petrinovich and I had used in the previous study. I was delighted (and astonished) to find that the rats given post-training injections of strychnine made fewer errors and required fewer training trials to learn the correct maze path leading to a food reward.[4] Moreover, the enhancing effect found was greater with higher drug doses. Thus, the post-training drug injections enhanced memory.

But was my conclusion correct? Did the post-training drug injections enhance memory? The findings certainly offered strong evidence suggesting that they did. I thought (or at least wanted to conclude) that they did. In scientific work, of course, experimental findings cannot *prove* a hypothesis to be *correct*. They can, however, show hypotheses to be *incorrect*. Ideas gain credence as alternative interpretations are eliminated by critical evidence. Obviously, then, before I could conclude with any degree of assurance that the post-training drug injections enhanced memory, other possible interpretations of the findings had to be considered.

All experiments need to consider and guard against the

possible bias of the experimenter. In my experiment I used the conventional procedure of marking the drug bottles with codes, to be broken only after I had completed the experiment. Thus, as I did not know which animals received the drug solutions and which received the saline control solution, experimenter bias seemed highly unlikely as an alternative interpretation of the findings. What about the possibility that the drug injections given after training might have been rewarding? After all, some kinds of drugs are well known to be rewarding. Subsequent studies found that post-training injections of low doses of convulsant drugs do not affect learning if the drug injections are substituted for the food reward. Thus, a reward interpretation of the effects can be excluded. Another possibility is that the drug injected after training may not have been completely metabolized or excreted within twenty-four hours and, thus, might have directly affected performance on the day after the injection. Other findings excluded this possible interpretation. Stimulant drugs are most effective when administered shortly after training. As injections administered several hours after training – that is, closer in time to the testing – do not affect memory, it is highly unlikely that drugs injected shortly after training directly affect retention performance. Retrograde enhancement of memory is shown in the top half of figure 5 in chapter 3.

In subsequent years, the finding that post-training administration of drugs can enhance memory was replicated in many experiments conducted in many laboratories throughout the world and alternative hypotheses were excluded by experimental findings.[5] Thus, the conclusion that drugs can enhance memory consolidation is now strongly supported by extensive evidence. It turned out to be not such a bad idea after all.

Going places, doing things

Studies of drug enhancement of memory began with studies of maze learning; but we know that there are many kinds of learning tasks, and that different tasks assess different forms of memory that engage different brain systems. So, without further evidence, the conclusion offered above may be somewhat too strongly stated. There is little doubt that drugs can enhance memory for food-rewarded maze training; but can they enhance memory for other kinds of tasks that may engage different brain systems than those used in maze learning? That important question has been asked, experimentally, in two ways. Many experiments have studied the effects of post-training administration of drugs on memory for many kinds of learning tasks typically used in studies of learning in animals, especially studies using rats and mice. These experiments make no special effort to determine that the tasks assess any specific memory or brain system; but such studies have used a variety of tasks that seem to provide a broad assessment of different kinds of learning that most likely rely on several brain systems. Other studies have used learning tasks thought to assess relatively specific forms of memory that engage specific brain systems. I will discuss some examples of both kinds of experiments. It is important to know at least a little about the types of tasks typically used in order to understand how the findings of studies using these tasks provide evidence of drug-enhancement of memory consolidation.

In mazes, animals clearly learn to go to specific places in the maze and, as training progresses, also learn to make responses, such as a sequence of turning responses. In view of the evidence (see chapter 2) that the hippocampus is engaged in the early stages of maze learning and the caudate nucleus later on, drugs administered after training may well affect both place and response learning. As is discussed later, there is ample evidence for this; but there is also clear evidence that drugs can enhance memory of *where*, in a maze, a reward was received on but a single training trial. In an early study of this issue,[6] Petrinovich and I trained thirsty rats in an open (i.e. with no walls) T-maze elevated about a metre above the floor. On each training trial they found water at the end of one alley of the maze. They were then taught that, on each succeeding trial, water reward was available only at the end of the *other* alley of the T. The only way for the animal to perform successfully was to remember the last choice made and then go to the other (i.e. opposite) alley on the next trial. Rats given an injection of saline after the initial trial could perform successfully on the next trial (i.e. select the other alley) even after a delay of about three hours. Rats given an injection of strychnine after the initial trial performed correctly on the next trial even with a delay of nine hours, or possibly even longer, as that was the longest delay tested. Clearly, memory of the place was enhanced, and not the response, because the correct choice required making a different response (right or left turn at the choice point of the T) from that made on the previous trial. In other experiments using an alley Y-maze, mice were given several food-reward training trials each day. The position of two alleys of the maze, one black and one white, was randomly shifted from left to right, and the mice were taught that the food was associated with the brightness of the alley, not the location. Low doses of several stimulant drugs enhanced retention when administered either immediately after each daily training session or within about an hour *after* or *before* the training sessions.

The type of reward or motivation used in training does not appear to be critical in studies of drug enhancement of memory. Many studies – perhaps most – use footshock for aversive training. Many experiments have used active avoidance tasks in which the animals are trained to make a particular response, such as shuttling from one side of a box to the other, pressing a lever, or turning a wheel in response to a signal in order to avoid a footshock. Such tasks clearly require the learning of what to do at the onset of a cue. In other experiments, animals are trained to discriminate between two cues, such as a dark or lighted alley, in order to escape from a footshock. In this task the animals learn what to do, i.e. escape, and where to go, i.e. a specific alley. Another task commonly used is contextual fear conditioning. In this task, animals are simply placed in an apparatus and given a series of footshocks. Memory of the training

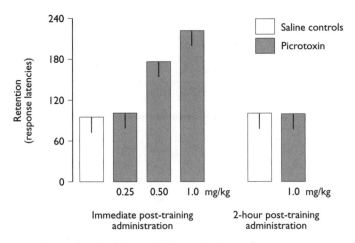

Figure 7 Picrotoxin administered after training enhances memory consolidation. Administration of this drug to rats immediately after inhibitory avoidance training produces an enhancement of memory tested a day later varying directly with the dose. Administration two hours after training does not affect memory. The post-training time-dependent effect is essential in allowing the conclusion that the drug influences memory consolidation. From Castellano and McGaugh, 1989.

experience is typically assessed by measuring the amount of time for which the animals freeze (i.e. remain immobile) when they are subsequently replaced in the apparatus.[7]

The aversive task that is perhaps most often used in studying memory enhancement is inhibitory avoidance, a task that has features in common with contextual fear conditioning.[8] For inhibitory avoidance training, animals are placed in a small starting compartment or on a small platform and receive a single low-intensity footshock after entering a larger compartment or stepping down from the platform. Memory of the one-trial training experience is usually tested a day or two later by replacing the animals in the starting compartment or on the platform and recording the length of the delay before they move to the place where they received footshock. The effects of one stimulant drug, picrotoxin, on inhibitory avoidance memory are shown in figure 7. Picrotoxin administered immediately after training enhanced retention performance tested the following day. An injection administered two hours after training did not affect memory.[9] These findings are similar to those of previous studies using maze learning tasks. Many studies by the British neuroscientist Steven Rose have studied memory enhancement in day-old chicks trained in a different type of inhibitory avoidance task.[10] The chicks are first allowed to peck at a bead dipped in a nasty-tasting solution. When the bead is presented to them the next day, they avoid the bead and their behaviour (I'm tempted to say, their facial expression) clearly suggests that they remember the nasty taste. For all types of inhibitory avoidance tasks, long delays in responding on the test are considered as evidence of good retention of the aversive experience. Also, as the learning occurs during a brief experience on a single training trial, it seems clear that the animals acquire and retain explicit information of the association between the training cues and the aversive experience.

Very clearly, drug enhancement of memory consolidation is not restricted to studies using maze learning. All of the tasks and procedures described above, as well as several others, have been used in studies of the enhancing effects of post-training drug administration on memory consolidation and evidence of memory enhancement has been found with all of these tasks.[11] Of course, we do not know that drugs can enhance the consolidation of memory for each and every possible kind of experience. There may well be memory for some kind or kinds of experience that is not enhanced by post-training drug administration; but there is now sufficient evidence to justify the strong conclusion that drugs can enhance memory consolidation and that the effect is not limited to specific types of memory or to a narrow range of memory tasks.

Selective significance

What, you might ask (and may well have asked while reading the discussion above), is the importance of knowing that drugs can enhance memory consolidation? It is highly doubtful that such findings will (or should) be put to use in animal training.

Imagine trying to give a post-training injection to an elephant or lion. Will such findings lead directly to the development of drugs for enhancing human memory? Will they cause the creation of little pills for the children's (or adults') lunch box? Unlikely. Is it important to know that memory can be enhanced? Not necessarily. But it *is* important to know that drugs administered immediately *after* training can enhance memory and that drugs administered several hours after training do not enhance memory – that is, the evidence that drugs can *selectively* enhance memory for *recent* experiences is the finding of critical importance.

Immediately after learning, the brain is in a state that allows either disruption (retrograde amnesia) or enhancement of the consolidation of long-term memory. These findings suggest two major questions (at least). First, why are our brains designed to allow such influences? That important issue, a major theme of this book, is addressed in the next chapter. Second, can we use information from studies of drug enhancement of memory to learn about brain mechanisms regulating memory consolidation? Let's consider that second question.

Flipping brain switches

Until now, I have discussed some effects of strychnine and picrotoxin, but have only vaguely referred to the memory-enhancing effects of other 'stimulants'. In the 1960s, many drugs with many different kinds of actions, including metrazol, physostigmine and amphetamine (as well as other drugs) were reported to enhance memory consolidation. The documented list is long; but the purpose of investigating many drugs is not to create a descriptive summary table. Different drugs affect the brain via different mechanisms. Each of the drugs mentioned above is now known to affect brain functioning in a different way. Understanding drugs' actions can suggest clues to the brain systems that consolidate memory. Let's consider what is known about several drugs. In order to discuss this research I

Table 1: Some drugs found to affect memory consolidation

Drug	Neuroreceptor action
Picrotoxin and Bicuculline	Blocks GABA receptors (GABA is an inhibitory neurotransmitter)
Diazepam (Valium)	(a benzodiazepine) Potentiates GABA effects
Flumazenil	Blocks benzodiazepine actions
Muscimol	Activates GABA receptors
Naloxone	Blocks opiate receptors
Morphine and Beta-Endorphin	Activates opiate receptors
Oxotremorine	Activates cholinergic receptors
Physostigmine	Acts indirectly to activate cholinergic receptors
Scopolamine and Atropine	Blocks cholinergic receptors
Amphetamine	Stimulates (indirectly) noradrenergic and dopaminergic receptors

have to use the names of quite a few drugs and indicate their major actions; table 1, which summarizes the effects of some of these on brain activity and memory consolidation, may be helpful in navigating the following sections.

In the early years of studies of drug effects on memory consolidation (late 1950s and early 1960s) little was known about the drugs' mechanisms of action. Strychnine, metrazol (pentylenetetrazol) and picrotoxin were known only as stimulants or convulsants. Metrazol was used, as discussed in chapter 2, to induce seizures in treating mental disorders and in investigation of drugs for treating epilepsy. In more recent decades much has been learned about how these and many other drugs that affect memory consolidation influence brain activity. The drug picrotoxin is now known to block the action of GABA (gamma amino butyric acid) a neurotransmitter in the brain that inhibits neuronal activity. Thus, the stimulation produced by picrotoxin is due *indirectly* to the blocking of receptors located on neurons that are activated by GABA released within the brain: inhibition of inhibition produces excitation. The drug muscimol, which acts like normally released GABA to inhibit neuronal activity, produces retrograde amnesia. Valium and other benzodiazepines used for treating anxiety act by increasing GABA-inhibitory effects. Thus, it is not surprising that such drugs impair memory consolidation[12] and that a drug (flumazenil) that blocks benzodiazepine actions enhances memory consolidation.[13]

Post-training injections of the excitatory neurotransmitter glutamate enhance memory, and drugs that block a specific type of receptor activated by glutamate impair memory. Drugs affecting the neurotransmitter acetylcholine also influence memory. Several drugs used to treat Alzheimer's disease prolong the actions of acetylcholine released by brain neurons by inhibiting an enzyme that degrades the acetylcholine. A drug that has this action, physostigmine, was among the first of several drugs found to enhance memory consolidation.[14] Such drugs thus produce stimulation of brain receptors (termed cholinergic receptors) sensitive to acetylcholine. Drugs such as oxotremorine directly stimulate one common type of cholinergic receptors (muscarinic) and drugs such as atropine and scopolamine block muscarinic cholinergic receptors. Many experiments have found that drugs that stimulate cholinergic receptors enhance memory and drugs that block such receptors produce retrograde amnesia.

A similar pattern of effects is found with several other classes of drugs – those, such as naloxone, that block opiate receptors enhance memory consolidation. The opioid peptide ß-endorphin and morphine, a drug that directly stimulates opiate receptors, impair memory consolidation. Drugs, such as amphetamine, that *indirectly* stimulate the receptors normally activated by norepinephrine (NE) (and dopamine, DA), as well as drugs that directly stimulate norepinephrine receptors (adrenoceptors), enhance memory consolidation, and drugs that block brain adrenoceptors can impair memory consolidation.

Thus, the story is a clear and consistent one: turning specific brain receptors on or off can affect memory consolidation; drugs that stimulate specific brain receptors and drugs that block those receptors have opposite effects on memory consolidation.[15]

Some sites to remember: almonds, sea horses and tails

The studies summarized briefly above were not, of course, obtained in order to create tables full of findings. Rather, the studies provide interesting and important evidence revealing how drugs act on some of the brain's communication chemicals, neurotransmitters (and *neuromodulators*, which regulate the actions of excitatory and inhibitory neurotransmitters) to influence memory consolidation. Most of the drugs mentioned above directly enter the brain shortly after they are injected systemically (i.e. into a vein, muscle or other peripheral body region), and it is there, in the brain, that they act to regulate the formation of lasting memory; but that conclusion, based on the summarized evidence, is but an inference. It seems safe to say that few of us would conclude that the drugs affect memory processes occurring *within* blood vessels, muscles or body cavities. The presumption that the drugs act in the brain can be examined by injecting drugs directly into specific regions of the brain. Many studies investigating this issue have found that all of the drugs discussed above affect memory consolidation when injected into specific brain regions; but, more interestingly, the drug effects obtained depend on the specific brain region that receives the drug injection. Thus, drugs are highly useful as tools in determining the involvement and role(s) of different brain regions in memory consolidation.

Almonds

The amygdala, an almond-shaped (in humans) region located on both sides of the brain deep within the temporal region, was one of the first brain regions studied in memory consolidation research (see figure 3, chapter 2). In the early 1960s Graham Goddard discovered that, in rats, electrical stimulation of the amygdala produced retrograde amnesia for an aversive training experience. Many subsequent studies confirmed these findings and found, additionally and importantly, that low-intensity stimulation of the amygdala after training *enhanced* memory.[16]

These studies firmly established the amygdala as a key brain site involved in memory consolidation.

These findings also suggested the interesting possibility that drugs injected directly into the amygdala might influence memory consolidation. In pioneering studies, Michela Gallagher and her colleagues found that a very small volume of low doses of the opiate receptor blocker naloxone, injected into the amygdala immediately after inhibitory avoidance training, enhanced rats' memory.[17] Injections of the opiate drug levorphanol impaired memory. They also found that intra-amygdala injections of drugs affecting adrenoceptors influenced memory consolidation. Subsequently, experiments in my laboratory studied the effects of several other drugs administered into the amygdala after inhibitory avoidance training, as well as other kinds of tasks mentioned above.[18] As we previously found with systemically injected drugs, intra-amygdala injections of the cholinergic stimulants physostigmine or oxotremorine enhanced memory, and injections of the cholinergic receptor blockers atropine or scopolamine impaired memory. Similarly, when injected into the amygdala after training, the GABA receptor antagonist bicuculline enhanced memory, and the GABA receptor antagonist muscimol impaired memory.

A clear picture appeared to emerge: for all drugs studied, systemic injections and injections into the amygdala produced comparable effects on memory consolidation; but additional studies revealed a more complex and interesting picture. Injections of adrenoceptor blockers (such as the beta blocker propranolol) into the amygdala prevented the memory-enhancing effects of bicuculline or naloxone. These findings suggested that these drugs influence memory, at least in part, through actions within the amygdala, and that the actions on memory require the triggering of adrenoceptors within the amygdala.

Thus, the complexity of the findings suggests simplicity in the *outcome* of drug actions in the amygdala. The influences of several kinds of drugs on memory consolidation appear to be integrated within the amygdala through the sum of their actions on the release of the neurotransmitter norepinephrine and activation of adrenoceptors. These findings and conclusions based on studies using drugs are also supported by studies using rats to examine the effects of drugs and training on the release of norepinephrine in the amygdala. These experiments used a microdialysis probe that was inserted into the amygdala to sample extracellular fluid. The fluid was then analysed to measure norepinephrine (using a technique called 'high-performance liquid chromatography', or HPLC). Systemically administered injections of naloxone or picrotoxin, drugs that enhance memory consolidation, increased norepinephrine levels. Drugs that impair consolidation, including muscimol, decreased norepinephrine release. In addition, and very interestingly, inhibitory avoidance *training* increased norepinephrine release in the amygdala. Furthermore, the subsequent retention performance of individual animals varied directly with the norepinephrine levels assessed in the amygdala after they were trained.[19] Clearly, norepinephrine released in the amygdala is an important regulator of memory consolidation (see table 2).

There is yet another interesting and important complexity. Injections of the cholinergic receptor blockers atropine or scopolamine into the amygdala prevent the memory-modulating effects of systemic *or* intra-amygdala injections of drugs acting

Table 2: Treatment effects on memory consolidation and amygdala norepinephrine release

Treatment	Neuroreceptor effect	Memory effect	Amygdala norepinephrine
Epinephrine	Adrenoceptor agonist	Enhances	Increases
Picrotoxin	GABAergic antagonist	Enhances	Increases
Muscimol	GABAergic agonist	Impairs	Decreases
Naloxone	Opiate receptor antagonist	Enhances	Increases
Beta-endorphin	Opiate receptor agonist	Impairs	Decreases
Inhibitory avoidance training			Increases

on opiate, GABA or adrenoceptors. Thus, integration of drug effects within the amygdala known to involve norepinephrine is also regulated by cholinergic stimulation within the amygdala. As will be discussed further in the next chapter, a particular sub-region of the amygdala, the basolateral amygdala, is the critical region involved in regulating memory consolidation.

Sea horses and tails

Do the drugs act only in the amygdala to influence memory? The answer to that is a clear no. Drugs can enhance memory when injected into several other areas after training. As we have already seen, many brain regions are given names based on their appearance. You can guess what the 'red nucleus' or the 'inferior olive' look like. Two regions important for memory, the hippocampus (sea horse) and caudate (tail) nucleus, were discussed briefly in previous chapters. Post-training injections of drugs into these brain regions also influence memory consolidation; but these regions care a lot about the *type* of information recently learned. Drug injections administered into these two regions *selectively* affect the consolidation for different kinds of training.

First, a little background. Many studies of this issue train rats in a 'Morris water maze',[20] which is simply a tank of water about six feet (or two metres) in diameter. In one task commonly used, rats are trained to swim to a slightly submerged (but not visible) clear plastic escape platform located in a specific *place* in the tank, using clearly visible 'landmarks', such as cabinets and posters located on the walls throughout the room. In another task they are trained to swim to a visible or 'cued' escape platform, with a patterned ball mounted on top of it, that is placed in a *different* location on each training trial. Experiments by Norman White and his colleagues, including Mark Packard,[21] found that brain damage affecting hippocampal functioning impaired rats' learning of the location of the submerged platform but did not affect learning to swim to the cued platform. In contrast, lesions of the caudate nucleus impaired the cued learning but not the place learning. Many studies investigating the effects of brain lesions have found that the hippocampus and caudate are selectively involved in different kinds of learning: place learning or cued learning (where to go or what to do). Thus, it was perhaps not surprising to learn, as Mark Packard and his colleagues subsequently did, that drugs injected into these two brain regions had different effects when injected after training in either place or cued learning. Amphetamine injected into the hippocampus post-training selectively enhanced memory for place training, and amphetamine injected into the caudate nucleus selectively enhanced memory for cued training.[22]

These two brain regions obviously have different jobs to do when faced with different learning tasks; but what do they do when faced with a task that enables learning both where to go *and* what to do? The study investigating the involvement of the hippocampus and caudate nucleus in learning in a T-maze discussed in chapter 2 found that the early stage of learning of the location of the reward involved the hippocampus and that continued training engaged the caudate nucleus in response learning. Mark Packard found that both kinds of learning in a T-maze could be enhanced by post-training injections; but the effect depended on which brain region, hippocampus or caudate nucleus, received post-training injections.[23] In this study rats received injections of a saline solution or the excitatory neurotransmitter glutamate administered into either the hippocampus or caudate nucleus each day, for several days, immediately after training. The reward was always located in the same place in the T-maze. On the eighth and sixteenth days they were tested, with the starting alley of the T-maze rotated 180 degrees in the room, to find out whether they had learned to go to a place in the room or make a turning response. Consistent with previous findings, the saline-control animals went to the *place* where they had received reward (making an opposite turning response) on Day 8 and on Day 16 made the *response* (left or right turn at the choice point in the T-maze) previously made on all training trials. Very different results were found with rats given the post-training drugs injections. Rats given glutamate injections into the hippocampus after each of the early training trials went to the *place* on both Day 8 and Day 16. They *maintained* place-going and did not, as the saline control rats did, shift to response learning with the additional training. Thus, the hippocampal injections of glutamate enhanced the rats' memory of the location of the reward and that memory remained strong despite additional training that would otherwise produce response learning. In contrast, rats given glutamate injections into the caudate nucleus after the early learning trials displayed response learning on Day 8 as well as Day 16. Activating the caudate nucleus after each early training trial enhanced response learning and accelerated the shift to response learning.

Almonds reprise

Clearly, some brain regions are dedicated to consolidation of specific kinds of information. The amygdala is promiscuous: in its influence on memory consolidation the amygdala appears not to care much, if at all, about the *kind* of information that is learned. This is perhaps not too surprising, as the amygdala is richly connected to many brain regions known to be involved in memory (see figure 8).[24] As noted above, drugs injected into the amygdala after training can enhance the long-term memories of many different kinds of training experiences. Experiments by Mark Packard, Larry Cahill and colleagues (see reference 22) showed quite clearly that the amygdala influences both *place* and *cued* learning. On the other hand, the experiments described above, in which rats were trained in place and cued water-maze tasks, confirmed that amphetamine injected into the hippocampus after training selectively enhanced place learning, and that injections administered into the caudate nucleus selectively enhanced cued learning. In contrast to the selectivity found with these two brain regions, post-training injections of amphetamine administered into the amygdala enhanced both place and cued learning.

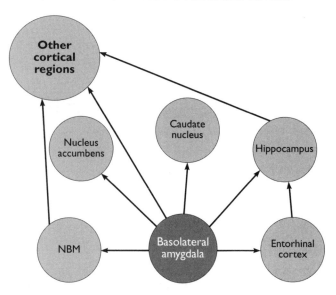

Figure 8 The basolateral amygdala is directly connected to many brain regions involved in memory consolidation. Through these connections it is able to modify the consolidation of memories that involve those brain regions.

These findings strongly suggest that the amygdala influences memory consolidation processes mediated by the hippocampus and caudate nucleus. Other findings of that study provided additional evidence supporting this conclusion. Injections of lidocaine into the hippocampus, to produce temporary inactivation of that brain region, completely prevented the enhanced place memory induced by amphetamine injected into the amygdala. Lidocaine injected into the caudate nucleus prevented the amygdala influence on cued learning. One other finding was of special importance: lidocaine injected into the amygdala before the test for memory of the place or cued learning did not impair memory. The memory for the training was very clearly not located in the amygdala.

Drugs administered to the amygdala appear to affect memory by altering the amygdala's influence on *other* brain regions involved in memory consolidation. It may even be that amygdala activity is *critical* in allowing the regulation of memory consolidation in other brain regions. Destruction of the stria terminalis, the neural pathway connecting the amygdala to the caudate nucleus, blocks the memory enhancement produced by post-training injections of a drug directly into the caudate nucleus.[25] Other studies from my laboratory found that lesions or temporary inactivation of the amygdala block the memory-enhancing effects of post-training injections of drugs into the hippocampus or the entorhinal cortex, a region of the cortex known to communicate directly with the hippocampus.[26]

In an extensive series of experiments using inhibitory avoid-ance training, Ivan Izquierdo and his colleagues[27] obtained addi-tional evidence indicating that the amygdala has only a temporary role in influencing memory. Infusions of drugs, such as muscimol, that inhibit neuronal activity, do not affect rats' retention performance when administered into the amygdala or hippocampus prior to retention tests one or two months after training. In contrast, such drug infusions impair retention per-formance when administered into the entorhinal cortex, or another cortical region, the parietal cortex, even two months after training. These findings strongly suggest that these corti-cal regions, unlike the amygdala and hippocampus, are brain sites that are critically involved in the long-term consolidation maintenance of lasting memory.

Drugs and lingering memories

Yes – to answer a question raised in the introduction to this chapter – drugs can enhance memory. Drugs with many kinds of actions enhance memory. The evidence considered here clearly indicates that drugs can enhance memory by stimulating the consolidation of memories of recent experiences. In providing this evidence, the studies of drug effects on memory consolida-tion have revealed some important clues to the mechanisms responsible for creating lasting memories. They led to the discov-ery that norepinephrine actions in the amygdala play an especial-ly important role. They have also identified the amygdala as a

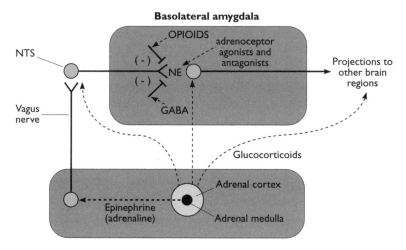

Figure 9 Stress hormone effects and neuromodulatory interactions occurring within the basolateral amygdala. Emotional arousal releases epinephrine (adrenaline) from the adrenal medulla and cortisol (corticosterone in the rat) from the adrenal cortex. Epinephrine activates receptors on the vagus nerve that connects in the brain to neurons that release norepinephrine (NE) in the amygdala. Cortisol passes freely into the brain, where it acts in many regions to influence memory consolidation. Release of NE and activation of noradrenergic receptors in the amygdala are critical in enabling the actions of cortisol. The inhibitory neurotransmitter GABA and opioid peptides inhibit the release of NE within the amygdala. Drugs that block the actions of GABA (e.g. picrotoxin) and opioid peptides increase NE release in the amygdala and enhance memory consolidation.

brain region that regulates memory consolidation by influencing other brain regions, including the cerebral cortex (see figure 9).

To sleep, perchance to dream

We spend about one third of our lives asleep. With current life expectancies, we can all expect to sleep for about twenty-five years. That's a lot of sleeping. Why do we do that? While we sleep each night, we dream. We accumulate a lot of years of dreaming time. In our dreams we do things and go places that are not beyond our wildest dreams because they *are* our wildest dreams. Despite the extensive and sustained efforts of generations of psychologists and neuroscientists, the causes and functions of sleep and dreaming are not yet known. Although we are generally poor at remembering our dreams, we have all experienced dreams that incorporate recent experiences, albeit in perhaps distorted and bizarre ways. Sleeping and dreaming must have at least some adaptive use if we are caused to spend so much time in those obscure states of mind.

One possible use of sleep, first suggested (to my knowledge) in 1925 by the psychologists J. G. Jenkins and K. M. Dallenbach,[28] is to prevent, or at least retard, forgetting. They found that memory of nonsense syllables tested after eight hours of intervening sleep was significantly better than that tested after eight hours of waking activity. So does sleep simply prevent the interfering effects of new learning? No: prior research by the German psychologist R. Heine in 1914[29] suggested that sleep acts in some way to promote the consolidation of recently learned material. Subjects learned lists of syllables either early in the evening or just before retiring to bed and were tested twenty-four hours later. The subjects who learned the material just before sleeping remembered the material better.

Those intriguing findings were allowed to consolidate, and languish, for many decades. In the mid-1900s, the studies of retrograde amnesia and memory consolidation reignited interest in examining the role of sleep in memory consolidation. Animal studies were the first to renew the inquiry. As assessed by EEG recordings of brain activity, there are two stages of sleep: slow-wave (low frequency, high amplitude) and REM (fast waves of low amplitude occurring with rapid eye movements). In an early study, William Fishbein (then a postdoctoral researcher in my laboratory) found that, in mice, retrograde amnesia was induced at an interval as long as two days after inhibitory avoidance training if the animals were deprived of REM sleep during that interval.[30] Subsequently, Vincent Bloch and his colleagues in Paris reported that REM sleep increased immediately after daily training on a maze and that REM

deprivation after training retarded the learning.[31] Those findings, too, appeared to require extensive consolidation as intense
interest in the role of sleep stages in memory consolidation has
emerged only in recent years.

Robert Stickgold and his colleagues[32] reported that human
subjects' improvement on a visual discrimination task occurred
only after the subjects had had a night's sleep and that, most
interestingly, the improvement varied directly with the amount
of slow-wave sleep during the early hours of sleeping and with
the amount of REM sleep occurring in the few hours before
waking. These findings strongly support Heine's hypothesis
that processes occurring during sleep, and not the passage of
time, are responsible for the consolidation of the memory of the
visual discrimination training. They also found that, with no
additional training, further improvement in performance occurs
after a second night's sleep; but that improvement requires the
first night's sleep. Sleep also promotes the consolidation of
motor skills. Jan Born and his colleagues found that eight hours
of sleep following practice on a finger-tapping motor skill
greatly improved subsequent performance on the task. These
findings strongly suggest that sleep is essential for consolidation of perceptual and motor skills. These findings may well
have important practical implications. Born and his colleagues
suggest: 'In generalizing these observations to skills of everyday
life (such as learning a musical instrument or sport) we would
conclude that sleep is required to achieved optimum performance on any of these skills.'[33] The fact that my high-school and
college band and orchestra rehearsals were typically scheduled
early in the morning of the school day may help explain (one
reason among a great many) why it is that I did not become a
professional musician. However, in developing such a skill it is
clear that, although sleep may be necessary, it is clearly not
sufficient!

The findings of these animal and human studies are clear and
consistent: sleep promotes memory consolidation; but what
processes occurring during sleep are responsible for these

effects? Bruce McNaughton and Matthew Wilson[34] reported that hippocampal neurons that were activated together in a pattern when animals were in a particular place in an apparatus during the daytime tended to fire together in the same pattern during subsequent sleep. Such patterned reactivation may, they suggested, play a role in consolidating memory of the previous day's experience. As the amygdala plays an important role in memory consolidation, it is not surprising that amygdala activation during sleep may be critical in the effects of sleep on memory consolidation. Denis Paré and his colleagues[35] have suggested that synchronized oscillations of the firing of amygdala neurons during sleep may facilitate the interactions between temporal lobe brain regions and the cortex essential for memory consolidation. The amygdala appears not to get much, if any, rest in regulating memory consolidation.

Rediscovering a role for the amygdala in memory

In science as well as other areas of human endeavour, important ideas often appear before their time and are neglected until findings encourage their 'rediscovery'. I recently discovered a prescient passage in a chapter by the neurophysiologist Ralph Gerard published decades before the studies of drug effects on amygdala functioning in memory were even dreamed of. Gerard suggested that the amygdala may act '...directly on cortical neurons to alter...their responsiveness to the discrete impulses that reach the cortex...these nuclei could easily modify the ease and completeness of experience fixation even if the nuclei were not themselves the loci of engrams.'[36] Of course, considerable evidence now supports his suggestion: the amygdala does appear to do just that. In the next chapter, I consider the significance of it being able to do so.

5 | Memorable Moments

'I remember numerous little "nothings" that I can remember of no other particular day...it is as if I were seeing this one day...through a pair of powerful glasses while I view the other days with just my own eyes, and see their events with almost a gray fog over them.'
REMEMBRANCE OF EVENTS OCCURRING BEFORE AN AUTO-MOBILE ACCIDENT – SIX YEARS EARLIER.[1]

'Remember when I fell at Kirby's house and cut my chin? I had this shirt on.'
SPONTANEOUS COMMENT OF MY TWO-AND-A-HALF-YEAR-OLD GRANDSON, TRISTAN ALVA, WHILE HIS MOTHER WAS PUTTING A SHIRT ON HIM. THE ACCIDENT HAD OCCURRED AT THE HOUSE OF HIS COUSIN (ANOTHER GRANDSON, KIRBY MORROW) ALMOST A YEAR EARLIER.

All memories are not created equal. I was at the front of a large room chairing a session at a scientific meeting in Portland, Oregon when someone came into the room and handed me a slip of paper. The message said simply that President Kennedy had been shot. I very clearly remember where I was and what I was doing when I received that message; but so do millions of other people who learned that the President had been shot on that November day in 1963; significant experiences create strong memories. As discussed briefly in a previous chapter, those witnessing horrific scenes, such as salvage debris from a plane crash in the ocean, typically say that the scene is something that will '...stick in their head for ever', or '...it is etched in my brain'. These kinds of comment are commonly found in newspaper and television interviews with those witnessing or experiencing calamities. Such statements appear to be correct. Testimonies of Nazi concentration camp prisoners obtained in 1943–7 and again in 1984–7 indicated that the horrific experiences of the camp were remembered in remarkably great and highly accurate detail over a period of forty years.[2] The expression 'etched' provides a woefully weak description of such strong memories; our most vivid memories die with us.

These reports and conclusions seem both obvious and valid. We all know from our own experiences that significant experiences are better remembered – or at least we think that we know that. Do I know for certain where I was and what I was doing when I learned that President Kennedy had been shot? If so, what specific details do I remember? Is my memory of that day more vivid than that of the day before or of a randomly selected day that year? What is it about that experience that may have caused it to be well remembered? Was it the uniqueness of my situation at the moment that the message arrived? Was it that the information was surprising? Was it my emotional response? Or, is my memory strong and accurate (if it is!) simply because I have thought about that event (i.e. rehearsed it) on many occasions in the intervening years? Although it may be possible to determine whether or not the details of an individual's experience are accurately remembered, determining *why* that is the case is not an easy matter. It would be relatively easy to find out whether my recollection summarized above is at least generally accurate. Was I where I remember being and was I doing what I remember I was doing at that time on that day? The programme of that meeting could be checked and those at the meeting could be interviewed. If my memory should turn out to be accurate, then we are left with the more important and difficult question: *why* do I remember the event of that day? Why is that memory privileged? To consider that question we need to examine the evidence from many who have investigated the conditions and brain processes that cause insignificant and significant experiences to create memories of different strengths. Let's first consider the conditions that create strong memories.

Vivid lasting memories of prominent public events

Many of our particularly significant experiences are shared by many. Those of us born before about 1955 no doubt remember, as I do, the announcement of President Kennedy's death. Other especially prominent public events remembered by many include such occurrences as the bombing of Pearl Harbor, the assassination of Martin Luther King, the explosion of *Challenger*, the resignation of Prime Minister Margaret Thatcher, the death of Princess Diana, the 1995 Oklahoma City bombing, major earthquakes and the planes crashing into the World Trade Center Towers in New York. Memory for events such as these has been extensively studied because the details of the events are explicitly known and the events themselves were immediately and widely known.

Are such events vividly remembered? This is the question that Roger Brown and James Kulik asked in their classic study of 'flashbulb memories'.[3] The term 'flashbulb memory' suggests that a memory of an event is preserved, much like a photograph, with clear, lasting details; but the analogy somewhat overstated the authors' intent. More generally, they suggested that such memories, though incomplete, contain details that are highly vivid and long-lasting. In their study they investigated subjects' memory of several public events (and one personally experienced event). The categories of recall used included where the subjects were, what they were doing, how they found out, personal emotional response at the time and personal consequences of the events. The public events that occurred years previously included the murders of Medgar Evers, John Kennedy, Malcolm X, Martin Luther King and Robert Kennedy as well as the attempted assassinations of George Wallace and Gerald Ford and the death of General Franco, the long-term dictator of Spain.

A central question was whether the 'consequentiality', or personal significance, of the event affected the reported memory of it. The evidence suggested that it did. Black subjects reported that they remembered more details about the deaths of

black public figures than did white subjects. In general, events
of less consequentiality, such as the attempted assassinations of
George Wallace and Gerald Ford and the death of General
Franco, were less well remembered. Equally, or perhaps more
importantly, the events that the subjects found highly surprising or shocking tended to be well remembered. As we will see
later, these findings provide some important clues to the
processes responsible for creating vivid and lasting memories of
public as well as personal events. Brown and Kulik discussed a
relatively specific neurobiological hypothesis in an attempt to
account for these findings; but before considering the neurobiological implications we need to consider some of the central
issues addressed in studies of flashbulb memory.

Are flashbulb memories *in fact* well remembered? Perhaps
surprisingly, this has been an issue of considerable (and heated)
debate. The debate and relevant evidence are very thoroughly and
thoughtfully discussed by Martin Conway in his comprehensive
book reviewing this topic, *Flashbulb Memories*.[4] We can first
dismiss an issue that concerns the specific characteristics of such
memories. The term 'flashbulb memory' is very clearly a mis-
leading one. Certainly, it should not be used if it is taken to mean
that such memories are complete and accurate in detail and that
the details of the events are not subject to any forgetting. The
issue is whether memories are especially strong, not whether
they are immutable. Second, and of course very importantly, are
such memories, in fact, accurate? We can, and certainly do, have
memories that are both strong and *inaccurate*. As we all know,
our family members and close friends are often joyously helpful
in noting and pointing out our mis-recollections. Any claim that
memory for significant public events is especially accurate must,
of course, be buttressed by evidence. Third, is personal consequentiality critical? Is it essential that the events have some personal significance or are surprising or shocking, perhaps
emotionally arousing? Prominent public events, however disastrous, may well have no particular personal significance. We do
not tend to remember where we were and what we were doing

when we learned that a severe and well-publicized earthquake occurred in Mongolia. Are our memories any different for nearby earthquakes or ones that we experience personally?

Let's first consider the issue of accuracy. We begin with an oft-cited report of strong and inaccurate personal memory of a public event that, paradoxically, provides evidence that significant memories are both accurate and durable:

> For many years I have remembered how I heard the news of the attack on Pearl Harbor...I recall sitting in the living room of our house...listening to a baseball game on the radio. The game was interrupted by an announcement of the attack...This memory has been so clear for so long that I never confronted its inherent absurdity until last year: no one broadcasts baseball games in December.[5]

Knowledge of another fact is required in order to understand the paradox. Charles Thompson and Thaddeus Cowan reported the following quote from an interview with the sportscaster Red Barber:

> I was at the Polo Ground to scout the New York Giants who... were to play the Chicago Bears...for the championship. I was to broadcast that game. The Giants were playing the old NFL football Dodgers. At half time, Lou Effrat of the New York Times came down from the press box and said Pearl Harbor had been bombed by Japan.[6]

Thus, the two *football* teams playing on 7 December 1941, the Giants and Dodgers (teams with the same names as those of two New York baseball teams), were playing in a well-known baseball field. Thus, it is perhaps not surprising that the game was remembered as a baseball game; and the event was vividly and otherwise very accurately remembered. Of course, such anecdotal evidence cannot settle the issue. We need to turn to evidence from studies of memory for significant public events.

The accuracy of self-reports of memories of public events is, at best, difficult to determine. It might be relatively safe to assume that self-reports are accurate if subjects are queried within a few days after the event – of course, reports given within hours would be even better – but such reports are not typically obtained. In place of *assured* accuracy, such studies typically investigate the *reliability* of the reported memories over time – that is, after a few months do the subjects provide the same answers to the questions concerning where they were, what they were doing, the emotions evoked, etc. as they gave shortly after the event? The evidence from several studies, including studies of memory of the *Challenger* disaster and of the assassination of the Prime Minister of Sweden, indicates that they *generally* do. Approximately fifty to ninety per cent of the responses given months, or even a year, after such specific events are similar to those given within a few days or weeks after the events.[7] Thus, the flashbulb memories of significant public events are relatively, not perfectly, stable. Again, such studies do not provide any clear evidence of their accuracy; other kinds of studies discussed below address that issue more extensively.

The reliability studies suggest that flashbulb memories do last over time – that they *are* strongly remembered – although the subjects in those studies may have been either consistently *poor* or consistently *good* at remembering the critical events shortly after learning and after a delay. However, other findings provide clear evidence that the details of significant public events are well remembered after delays of many months. Subjects who experienced the 1989 California earthquake (the epicentre was near Santa Cruz, California) recalled almost all of the details originally provided shortly after the earthquake when questioned again eighteen months later.[8] In contrast, subjects living in Georgia, who did not directly experience the earthquake, remembered many fewer details eighteen months after the earthquake. Similarly, subjects in England who were UK nationals had very strong and detailed memories of Prime Minister Thatcher's surprising resignation (in 1990) both two weeks after the event and eleven months later.[9] In contrast, subjects who were not UK nationals (mainly North Americans) were very poor at remembering the details on the eighteen-month test. Findings of these kinds of study support two conclusions: first, significant public events can be very well remembered after long delays; second, consequentiality is important. Subjects' personal reactions to the event, including emotional responses, appear to play a major role in influencing the strength of the memories.

Considerable evidence from many flashbulb memory studies supports the conclusion that emotional responses evoked by the event influence memory of the event. Subjects' reported emotional reactions appeared to contribute to their memory of the *Challenger* disaster as well as to their memory of the soccer match in England where ninety-five people were crushed to death (the 'Hillsborough disaster').[10] As noted above, emotional responses also influence memories of interesting and exciting but considerably less disastrous events. The O. J. Simpson murder trial in 1995 was the focus of considerable public attention. The trial was very highly publicized in the media and shown on television; there was wide and intense interest in the jury's verdict. Three days after the jury announced the highly controversial verdict of 'not guilty', Heike Schmolck, Elizabeth Buffalo and Larry Squire initiated a study of subjects' memory of when, where and how the subjects found out about the verdict as well as of the strength of their emotional reactions to it.[11] The questionnaire given to the subjects asked for many more details, including whether the subjects agreed or disagreed with the verdict and the extent to which they discussed it with others. Twenty-four per cent of the subjects agreed with the verdict, forty per cent disagreed with it and thirty-six per cent were neutral. The accuracy of the recollections was studied in two groups queried either fifteen months or thirty-two months later. When questioned fifteen months after the verdict, two-thirds of the subjects had recollections that were the same as the original responses or that were only minor distortions. Ten per cent of the subjects had major distortions in their recollections. The recollections of subjects tested at thirty-two months were less accurate. Although approximately fifty per cent had either no distortions or only minor distortions in their recollections, over forty per cent of the subjects had major distortions. Clearly, the accuracy of the recollections decreased over time; nonetheless, the memories remained reasonably, perhaps even surprisingly, strong over the thirty-two-month delay. The subjects' self-ratings shortly after the verdict provide some clues to the accuracy of the recollections assessed at thirty-two months. Accuracy was not associated with the amount of rehearsal of the details, interest in the trial, agreement with the verdict or the subjects' strength of opinion about the verdict. However, accuracy of recollection thirty-two months after learning the verdict was significantly associated with the intensity of their *emotional responses* when they learned the verdict.

Although memories of such significant public events may not be etched in our brains and stick there for ever, they do appear to be more vivid and long-lasting. Recollections of witnesses of violent crimes can be even more vivid and durable. John Yuille and Judith Cutshall[12] interviewed subjects who had witnessed a shop owner shoot and kill a man who had just robbed him. The interviews occurred either on the day of the crime or two days after the event and, for some subjects, four to five months later. Accuracy of their reports could be confirmed by considerable evidence obtained at the crime scene, from photographs, emergency services and medical reports. On both interviews, over eighty per cent of the subjects' recollections were accurate. Five of the twenty-one witnesses reported that they were highly stressed while witnessing the killing. The accuracy of these subjects was ninety-three per cent on the first interview and eighty-eight per cent on the second.

Stronger etching in the brain? It does appear so. All of the evidence reviewed above points to at least one general and important conclusion: emotionally significant events create stronger, longer-lasting memories. Whether subjects experience the events, witness them, hear about them on the radio, see them or reports about them on television, or learn about them from friends and neighbours, the events are likely to be recalled months or even years later; but, like memories of ordinary events, they are neither *completely* accurate nor, in all cases, *permanently* strong. Consider the twenty per cent of subjects whose recollections of the killing were inaccurate. Such mis-recollections could well be critical if the subjects served as witnesses in a trial. Flashbulb memories are not like photographs: they are not highly precise in detail and may change or fade over time. Moreover, we need to consider what we mean by a 'public event' or even a crime scene these days, when the events may be, and usually are, repeatedly shown on television and discussed in detail in newspapers, magazines and on the Internet. What is *the event* that is experienced? How often have we seen the film clip of President Kennedy's assassination? How many times has the *Challenger* catastrophe been shown on television? How frequently have we seen the wrecked car that Princess Diana was riding in when it crashed in the tunnel in Paris? How often have we seen the crumbling Twin Towers in New York? These repeated experiences can, and do, influence our memories of where we were and what we were doing when we *first* learned of an event. Do we remember the first time, the second time or some other time? Such repeated exposures and our repeated thinking about them ('rehearsal') no doubt contribute significantly to our mis-recollections of the original event and create a 'generic' memory of it. Perhaps somewhat surprisingly, however, such studies have provided very little evidence that rehearsal of the memory of the event is critical in creating a flashbulb memory. Nonetheless these several possible influences are often difficult to disentangle in flashbulb memory studies based on important and well-publicized events. Although the conclusions drawn from flashbulb memory studies seem well supported by the evidence, evidence from emotionally significant experiences that are not public events is needed to deal with the caveats just considered.

Back to the laboratory

As we know, Ebbinghaus taught us that extensive repetition strengthens our memory for words. Does emotional arousal also strengthen memory for something as simple (and boring?) as 'Ebbinghausian' word associations? Yes: evidence from many studies indicates that, as with memory for public events, emotional arousal enhances long-term memory for word associations learned in the laboratory. In a study that first triggered interest in this issue, L. Kleinsmith and S. Kaplan[13] had subjects learn to associate pairs of words. Some of the words in the pairs (e.g. 'kiss', 'vomit', 'rape') were used because they elicited strong emotional responses, as indicated by changes in the subjects' galvanic skin response (GSR), a commonly used measure of emotional arousal. On a retention test a week later the subjects remembered emotionally arousing words better than they remembered less arousing words. Interestingly, the emotionally arousing words were poorly remembered on tests given shortly after the learning; the enhanced memory was seen only after a delay. I'll consider some additional evidence concerning this latter issue later in this chapter.

One might question (and you may well have) the relevance of such findings for our memories of events in our lives. Well, perhaps a phone number just dialled might be well remembered if the call connects us to the Inland Revenue, or to someone who tells us that we have just won the lottery or that a loved one has survived a heart attack; but we are equally, or more, likely to remember other details concerning the telephone call: where it occurred, who answered, what happened just before and after the call. We remember details of events that occur over time. They do not have to be real events: they can be events in stories read or listened to, or movies. The success and remembrance of novels and movies depend heavily on their emotional content, as we all know. The scenes and storylines can combine to create powerful emotional responses.

What, though, is remembered if *different* storylines, one

emotional and one less emotional are associated with the same scenes? Does the level of emotional arousal induced by a story affect subjects' memory of what they see during the telling of the story? Larry Cahill and I asked this question[14] in an experiment using procedures and materials based on the seminal work of Friderike Heuer and Daniel Reisberg.[15] Subjects in two groups viewed exactly the same series of twelve slides. They were told only that the study concerned physiological responses to stimuli of different kinds. The slide presentation for each group was accompanied by a story – one sentence of the story for each slide. For one group, the narrative was relatively boring (or neutral): a mother and her son leave home to visit a hospital, where they watch disaster-drill procedures, and then the boy remains with his father while his mother leaves. For the other group, the narrative was emotionally arousing: after leaving home the boy is critically injured in an accident, is rushed to a hospital, where surgeons manage to re-attach his severed feet; the boy's father remains with him while his mother leaves. The narratives were identical only for the first four slides and the final slide. Subjects' ratings of the emotionality of the stories confirmed that they produced different levels of emotional arousal.

The subjects were asked to return in two weeks but were not told that this was a study of their memory. When they returned, they were tested for their memory of specific details in the slides they had seen. Subjects in the two groups did not differ in their recognition or recall of details in the first few slides or the last few slides. They did, however, differ in their remembrance of the content of the slides shown in the middle of the narration – where the stories differed in emotional impact. The subjects who had listened to the emotionally arousing narrative remembered details in those particular slides better. Those who had listened to the neutral story did not have better memory for those slides than they did for slides that came before or after them.

The slides presented during the most emotional part of the

story were, then, better remembered. Thus, these findings are consistent with those of flashbulb memory studies and memory for emotionally arousing words: stronger emotional arousal is associated with better memory; emotional arousal appears to create strong memories. 'Emotion provides no guarantee of permanent or perfectly accurate recall – emotional memories will contain errors...Nonetheless...we can largely trust our vivid memories of emotional events.'[16]

So the evidence from many kinds of studies is consistent, and the conclusion is that inducing emotional arousal is one way of creating stronger memory. We now need to know *why*. What are the consequences of emotional arousal that play roles in memory? Certainly, enhanced attention to the experiences during emotional arousal is one reasonable and likely possibility. As discussed above, emotional experiences may be rehearsed more often, either deliberately or inadvertently. Ebbinghaus has told us what rehearsal does; but although this possible interpretation seems reasonable, the evidence for an effect of rehearsal in accounting for the effects of emotional arousal on memory is not strong or convincing. Shannon Guy and Larry Cahill[17] investigated this issue explicitly, by studying subjects' memory for the content of neutral and emotionally arousing films one week after they had viewed them. After viewing the films, one group of subjects was instructed to refrain from discussing them. Another was instructed to discuss the films with at least three people. A third group was instructed not to talk about the films but admitted that they did not comply with the instructions. As was expected, all groups remembered the emotionally arousing films better than they did the neutral films. However, perhaps surprisingly, talking about the films, whether in response to the instructions or because of non-compliance with the instructions, did not affect the subjects' memory of the films. The findings do not mean, of course, that rehearsal *cannot* influence memory: we know that it can. The findings simply indicate that a modest amount of discussion of the films did not affect memory of them. Again, importantly, as in previous studies of many kinds, emotional arousal *did*, and we need to know why.

Making memorable moments

'Events previous to the time of my being struck by the train are in bold relief... the events of the five minutes previous [after three and a half years] are as any events two days past. I believe that I can account for every move of these five minutes. The time is completely filled in my memory.'[18]

Interest in the relationship between the significance of an event and its remembrance did not, of course, begin with studies of flashbulb memory. Comments similar to those quoted above were perhaps made by our ancestors as they were painting pictures of animals in caves in southern France. Who knows? Maybe that's why they painted those pictures. Exciting experiences recorded in the brain are worth recording in paintings.

Robert Livingston in 1967 was, to the best of my knowledge, the first to suggest some relatively specific brain mechanisms that might create such lasting and detailed memories. He proposed that:

...whenever something...is...highly meaningful...and significant... the associated remembrance includes even aspects which themselves are not pertinent to the meaningfulness of the occasion. The brain 'prints' remembrance of all events immediately preceding, regardless of whether the events have any real significance for the central matter involved.[19]

To account for the 'print' action Livingston proposed that the experiences activate the 'limbic' system (a collection of brain regions, including the amygdala, nestled toward the centre of the brain), which, in turn, stimulates the 'reticular activating system' that projects diffusely throughout the brain and provides a 'Now print!' order: 'Following a..."Now print!" order, everything that has been ongoing in the recent past will receive a "Now print!" contribution in the form of a growth stimulus or a neurohormonal influence that will favor future repetitions of the same neural activities.'

Four years later, Seymour Kety proposed a similar but somewhat more specific hypothesis suggesting that emotionally activated release of the neurotransmitter norepinephrine might facilitate consolidation at recently activated brain synapses and noted that '...there is obvious adaptive advantage in a mechanism that consolidates not all experiences equally'.[20]

So far I have reviewed some of the extensive evidence that emotional arousal influences long-term memory and very briefly discussed two closely related ideas (Livingston's and Kety's) about how the brain might make that happen. In scientific inquiry, the proposal of hypotheses and accumulation of relevant evidence don't always appear in that sequence. Sometimes critical evidence appears first; and, sometimes relevant *suggested* experiments are discovered only after the experimental evidence is available. The evidence that drugs administered after training can enhance memory consolidation was first obtained in my laboratory during the late 1950s and first published in 1961, several years before Livingston and Kety offered their hypotheses. The findings reviewed in chapter 4 provided extensive evidence that many drugs can enhance memory consolidation. Drugs administered immediately after training experiences enhanced memory of the experiences; drugs administered several hours later did not. Quite clearly, the evidence from many studies published in the early 1960s indicates that drugs such as strychnine, picrotoxin and amphetamine, as well as many other stimulant drugs, act on learning-induced neural processes that continue after the learning experience.[21] They make significant events more memorable. Did the drugs trick the brain into activating the 'Now print!' signal? Do they work by activating specific brain systems that have widespread influence on brain activity? Does norepinephrine play a role? The answer appears to be yes to all of the above; but there is much more to the story.

Nothing like a little stress

My first studies of the memory-enhancing effects of post-training drug injections were conducted when I was a graduate student. My research advisor, David Krech, who, as I noted earlier, spent the year in Europe while I conducted those studies, agreed on his return that it was not such a bad idea after all. He then discussed the findings briefly at an international meeting. One of the scientists present at that meeting, the eminent neurophysiologist Ralph Gerard, quickly saw the physiological implications. He wrote:

> Strychnine according to an informal communication from Dr. Krech, shortens fixation time … Any change that would enhance the extent or intensity of reverberation should hasten the fixation process … Since epinephrine [adrenaline] … lowers (cortical) thresholds, and is released in vivid emotional experiences, such an intense adventure should be highly memorable.[22]

That prescient suggestion was, and remained (as scientific ideas often are), lost in the mists of time; but it turned out to be an interesting guess, as we shall see. Until the early to mid-1970s research investigating drug influences on memory consolidation continued to study the kinds of drugs that were effective and the forms of learning and memory susceptible to post-training enhancement. The research was not explicitly – or perhaps even implicitly – linked to the issue of emotion and memory. In retrospect, that was an obvious issue that we, and others working in this area of research, had overlooked.

Our interest shifted to that issue when we began to consider the important question of why it is that we and many other species have brains that are so susceptible to influences occurring after an experience that induce retrograde amnesia or retrograde enhancement of memory. Do the drugs and other treatments used in such experiments simply cause brains to do things that they don't ordinarily do, or do the treatments tap

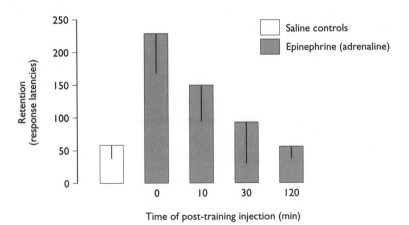

Figure 10 Epinephrine administered after training enhances memory consolidation. The effect varies with the interval between training and hormone administration. Administration two hours after training does not affect memory. From Gold and van Buskirk, 1975.

into and take advantage of some physiological system that regulates memory consolidation? It is important to note that a drug's influences on attention during learning can be excluded as an interpretation of post-training drug influences on memory consolidation, as the event is over when the drug is administered. By default (as well as by theoretical expectation), enhancement of processes underlying memory consolidation seems the only reasonable conclusion offered by the experimental findings.

At that time, Paul Gold (now a professor at the University of Illinois) was a postdoctoral researcher in my laboratory. What endogenous substances released or activated by training experiences, we asked, might have effects on memory like those induced by stimulant drugs administered after training? Many studies in our laboratory used footshock as part of the training. In particular, animals trained in an inhibitory avoidance task received a single footshock after stepping into a darkened alley. The use of these procedures suggested a reasonable possibility: perhaps, we thought, the stress hormones epinephrine (adrenaline) and cortisol (or corticosterone, in the rat) released from the adrenal gland after the animals received the footshock acted like stimulant drugs to modulate memory consolidation processes.

Gold and a graduate student in my laboratory, Roderick van Buskirk, investigated this possibility.[23] They administered a saline solution or epinephrine (in different doses) to rats either immediately after they were trained in the inhibitory avoidance task or at different times after the training. Retention of memory of the training was tested the next day. As is shown in figure 10, epinephrine administered immediately after training greatly increased the rats' memory of the training, as assessed by their reluctance to re-enter the alley where they had previously received a footshock. In addition, and equally importantly, the effectiveness of epinephrine in enhancing memory decreased with increasing delays in the time of the post-training injection. Providing a little more stress hormone after the learning experience produced a stronger memory of the experience. These findings suggested that stimulant drugs administered post-training most likely do tap into a physiological memory modulating system; and maybe Gerard's suggestion about epinephrine actions (see reference 22) was correct – but maybe not. We'll first have to consider some of the evidence from several other studies. Later on in this chapter we'll also have to consider the contribution of the other major adrenal stress hormone cortisol (corticosterone in rats).

First, a stumbling block called the 'blood–brain barrier'. Because of that barrier, epinephrine does not enter the brain freely, if at all. If epinephrine doesn't enter the brain, then, of course, it can't *directly* influence brain neuronal activity; but other findings of Gold and van Buskirk showed that, nonetheless, epinephrine does very significantly affect the brain. Epinephrine injected after inhibitory avoidance training produced a transient but significant increase (20–40%) in the release of brain norepinephrine.[24] The arousing effects of footshock alone also stimulated the release of brain norepinephrine.

Although it may seem more important to know *that* the brain was influenced than *how* epinephrine affected the brain, the question 'How?' is interesting and worth a brief discussion, as the findings bear on results of human as well as animal studies of emotionally influenced memory discussed below. Propranolol, a drug that blocks ß-adrenoceptors (a beta blocker) prevents the memory-enhancing effects of epinephrine. That is not a surprising finding, as propranolol injected into muscles or veins influences ß-adrenoceptors located outside the brain and also passes freely into the brain and blocks receptors there. However, another beta blocker, sotalol, which does not enter the brain, also blocks the memory-enhancing effects of epinephrine.[25] Thus, epinephrine effects on memory are initiated at least partly by activation of ß-adrenoceptors located *outside* the brain; but a body–brain connection is required.

One possibility – one that Gold has investigated extensively – is that epinephrine effects on memory may be mediated, in part, by releasing glucose from the liver.[26] Glucose, in turn, can enter the brain and directly affect neuronal functioning. In support of this hypothesis, he found that, like epinephrine, glucose administered post-training enhances memory consolidation; but epinephrine also affects the brain via another route. In a series of experiments, Cedric Williams (a postdoctoral researcher in my laboratory, now a professor at the University of Virginia) and others[27] showed that critical ß-adrenoceptor receptors are also located on the ascending vagus nerve that originates in the body and connects in a nucleus of the brain stem (the nucleus of the solitary tract, or NTS). Very interestingly, the NTS connects to the amygdala where it can, and does, release norepinephrine (see figure 9). The epinephrine that Gold and van Buskirk used (or that released by footshock) seemed to take advantage of this neural pathway into the amygdala; but we need to consider a little more evidence before drawing that conclusion firmly.

Almonds, sea horses and tail reprise

Let's first consider epinephrine influences on the amygdala. From the discussion in chapter 4, we know that several drugs that enhance memory consolidation also induce the release of norepinephrine in the amygdala and that the effects involve stimulation of ß-adrenoceptors in the amygdala; but is norepinephrine release within the amygdala critical for *epinephrine* effects on memory consolidation? Keng Chen Liang, a graduate student in my laboratory (now a professor at Taiwan National University), asked that question. The answer was yes. He discovered this by injecting a small amount of propranolol into the amygdala immediately after training, just before he injected epinephrine peripherally. The epinephrine injections alone would have enhanced memory; propranolol administered into the amygdala, however, blocked the epinephrine-induced memory enhancement.[28] Propranolol blocked the actions of norepinephrine released by epinephrine (via the vagus connection). Liang also found that post-training injections of norepinephrine administered into the amygdala enhanced memory consolidation. These findings confirmed those of Michela Gallagher[29] discussed in the previous chapter. This effect was subsequently replicated in many subsequent experiments using injections administered selectively into one sub-region of the amygdala, the basolateral amygdala.[30]

Equally importantly, Liang found that lesions of a major pathway connecting the amygdala to other brain regions (the stria terminalis, or ST) prevented the memory enhancement induced by norepinephrine administered into the amygdala post-training.[31] These results strongly suggested that the norepinephrine influenced memory via influences on other brain regions involved in memory consolidation. As discussed in chapter 4, amphetamine injected into the amygdala post-training influenced memory of a training experience known to involve the caudate nucleus. As the stria terminalis pathway connects the amygdala to the caudate nucleus, lesions of this pathway should block amygdala–caudate interactions in memory consolidation. Experimental findings support this implication. Lesions of the stria terminalis prevent the memory enhancement otherwise produced by injections of a drug (the cholinergic drug oxotremorine) administered into the caudate nucleus after training.[32]

All of the findings of epinephrine effects summarized above fit extremely well with the conclusions offered in chapter 4 (see figure 9). Norepinephrine released in the amygdala is very clearly an important regulator of memory consolidation; and the regulation very clearly involves influences on other brain regions involved in memory consolidation. But what about corticosterone, the other major stress hormone released from the adrenal gland into the bloodstream by even mildly stressful stimulation? Does it also play a role in memory consolidation? Yes, there is considerable evidence that post-training injections of corticosterone, as well as synthetic drugs with actions like that of corticosterone, enhance memory consolidation.[33] There is no blood–brain barrier stumbling block for this hormone to contend with, as it readily passes into the brain, where it activates glucocorticoid receptors *within* neurons in many brain regions; but, as with epinephrine, the amygdala is critical. Moreover, and very importantly, my research colleague Benno Roozendaal and I found, in an extensive series of experiments, that norepinephrine in the amygdala is critical. Propranolol and other ß-adrenoceptor blockers injected selectively into the amygdala (basolateral nucleus) prevent the memory-enhancing effects of drugs that, like corticosterone, stimulate glucocorticoid receptors.

Several decades ago, Bruce McEwen at Rockefeller University made the highly important and influential discovery that the hippocampus is densely populated with glucocorticoid receptors.[34] Thus, if that brain region is involved in some forms of memory (learning about events and places), perhaps activation of those receptors will influence memory consolidation. The evidence indicates that it does. Benno Roozendaal found that post-training injections of drugs that activate glucocorticoid receptors administered directly into the hippocampus enhance memory consolidation (see reference 33). Does this mean that the amygdala is not involved, or is not needed for this memory-enhancing effect? No, on the contrary. Lesions of the amygdala, or blocking of ß-adrenoceptors in the *amygdala*, prevent the memory enhancement otherwise produced by post-

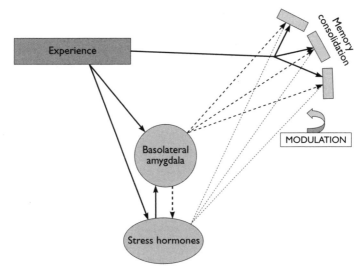

Figure 11 Interaction of stress hormones with the amygdala in modulating memory consolidation in other brain regions. Experiences initiate memory consolidation in many brain regions. Emotionally arousing experiences also activate the basolateral amygdala and the release of stress hormones (epinephrine and cortisol) from the adrenal gland. The stress hormones also activate the amygdala by influencing noradrenergic receptors in the basolateral amygdala. Neural projections from the amygdala to other brain regions modulate the memory consolidation occurring in those regions. Cortisol can directly modulate consolidation, but the modulation also requires amygdala activation concurrently.

training activation of glucocorticoid receptors selectively within the *hippocampus*. Again, the amygdala has a central and critical role in enabling and modulating memory consolidation processes in other brain regions (see figure 11).

Double-duty stress hormones

Thus, these two major adrenal stress hormones, epinephrine and cortisol, that have quite different ways (and pathways) of affecting the brain, have a common action in influencing norepinephrine functioning within the amygdala that is critical for modulating memory consolidation. These two stress hormones are very busy in helping us manage our lives. They have many important and complex duties to perform in helping us deal with the immediate physiological consequences of stressful events. They are part of our emergency 'first-aid' kit; but they both also do double duty. In addition to providing emergency physiological aid, they both also serve the highly important function of strengthening our memories of the stressful events that caused their release from the adrenal glands. Yes, there is nothing like a little stress to help create strong, long-lasting memories of events we have experienced.[35]

There is, however, an important and interesting caveat. The effects of stress on recalling previously learned information are yet another matter. Did you ever have the experience of 'blocking' in an exam, an interview, a court testimony, a public speech or even the reciting of a marriage vow? Well, most of us *have* had such experiences. They are *usually* real memory failures, not fabricated excuses for poor memory performance (of course, fabrication is also possible). In two experiments, Dominique de Quervain and Benno Roozendaal and their colleagues have shown that, in human subjects as well as rats, a brief stressful experience impairs retrieval of well-established memories.[36] The impaired retrieval lasts for about an hour. Additionally, they found that the retrieval impairment was due to the release of corticosterone (rats) or cortisol (humans) as it was blocked by a drug that prevents the synthesis and release of adrenal glucocorticoids. Thus, a little stress is not *always* good for memory – it can temporarily impair our ability to recall or retrieve even well-learned information. Although it is too late to correct your grade on an exam taken long ago, you may well wish you could inform the teacher who graded your exam that your poor performance was caused by your glucocorticoid receptors (maybe).

Emotional arousal, stress hormones, amygdala activation and human memory

Animal experiments have provided most of what we know

about the actions of drugs, hormones and the amygdala in regulating memory consolidation. The reason for this is obvious: animals can be trained in specific ways and given drugs or hormones at specific times and into specific regions of the brain after training. The use of post-training treatments excludes any influence on the animals' attention at the time of training. In addition, the animals' experiences during the delay before retention testing can be carefully controlled. Explicit rehearsal of the training experience by the animals seems, at best, unlikely. Well, *maybe* it is unlikely. Unfortunately, we can't know that for certain because we have no way of determining whether animals can explicitly rehearse their past experiences. Although experiments with human subjects have to use methods and experimental techniques quite different from those used in animal studies, the findings of many human studies of the effects of drugs, stress hormones and emotional arousal on memory are, nonetheless, highly consistent with those of animal studies.

A little more stress

In Larry Cahill's study discussed earlier in this chapter, reporting that emotional arousal selectively enhanced subjects' long-term memory of information in slides accompanying an emotionally arousing narrative, was the enhanced memory caused, at least in part, by stress hormone release? Evidence from subsequent experiments using the same materials and experimental procedures strongly suggests that it was. In a first study,[37] Cahill gave the beta blocker, propranolol, or a placebo pill to subjects just before they saw the series of slides accompanied by a neutral or emotionally arousing narrative. On a surprise memory test two weeks later, subjects given the placebo had enhanced memory for the content of the slides associated with the middle, emotionally arousing part of the narrative. In contrast, subjects given propranolol did not have enhanced memory for those slides. Thus, propranolol, which is known to block the actions of epinephrine and norepinephrine, prevented the effects of emotional arousal on memory. Propranolol did not impair memory of the slides associated with the non-emotional portions of the narrative and did not impair memory of the slides shown along with the neutral narrative. Other studies using the same general procedures confirmed those findings and found that yohimbine, a drug that stimulates norepineph-rine release, enhanced subjects' long-term (i.e. one week) memory of the content of the slides accompanied by the narra-tive.[38] In another study, using somewhat different experimental procedures, Kristy Nielson and Robert Jensen[39] found that arousal induced after reading narrative paragraphs increased elderly subjects' memory for paragraphs. However, and impor-tantly, arousal did not increase memory in elderly subjects who were taking beta blockers for treatment of hypertension. As dis-cussed above, epinephrine effects on memory are initiated, at least partly, by activation of beta receptors located on the ascending vagus nerve that connects with a nucleus in the brain stem that, in turn, projects to the amygdala, where it releases norepinephrine. In a very ingenious series of studies, Jensen and his colleagues found that direct electrical stimulation of the ascending vagus nerve after learning also enhances memory in human subjects (as well as in rats).[40] However, the vagus nerve brain connection is not the sole pathway that epinephrine uses to enhance memory. Epinephrine-induced release of glucose from the liver also appears to play a role. Gold and his col-leagues reported that glucose enhances memory consolidation in elderly adults, as well as in rats.[41]

Thus, the findings of experimental studies of human memory are quite consistent with those investigating memory in animals: arousal influences memory consolidation; and, perhaps most importantly, the influence is due, at least in part, to the release of epinephrine and norepinephrine and activation of ß-adrenoceptors. As with studies of memory in animals, acti-vation of glucocorticoid receptors also plays a central role. Buchanan and Lovallo[42] reported that cortisol given to subjects shortly before they viewed emotionally arousing pictures enhanced the subjects' memory of the pictures assessed one week later.

At this point you may ask what all of these experimental studies of stress hormone influences on memory have to do with memories of stressful events occurring in our lives. Studies of critically-ill hospital patients indicate that such studies are highly relevant in understanding traumatic memories. The majority of patients treated in a hospital intensive care unit typically have strong, long-lasting memories of their traumatic experiences including their nightmares, anxiety, respiratory distress or pain. Gustav Schelling and his colleagues, in Munich,[43] studied such traumatic memories in patients who had received cardiac surgery for heart disease or heart valve replacement and required intensive care therapy for many days or weeks. The treatment often includes administration of stress-level doses of epinephrine and hydrocortisone. When queried six months after such treatments, the strength of the patients' memories of the traumatic experiences varied directly with the administration of epinephrine and stress-level doses of hydrocortisone they received while being treated in the hospital. Higher doses of these stress hormones resulted in stronger long-term memories. Yes – to consider the question asked at the beginning of this paragraph – animal and human experiments investigating the memory-enhancing effects of adrenal stress hormones do appear to have clear relevance for understanding memories of stressful events in our lives.

The absent amygdala

Do the enhancing effects of arousal on human memory involve the amygdala? The findings of animal experiments certainly (and strongly) suggest that the amygdala is involved in mediating such effects; but in human studies the question has to be asked in very different ways from those of animal studies. Let's first consider the effects of lesions of the amygdala.

Several studies have investigated the effects of emotional arousal on memory in human subjects who have a very rare medical condition that can result in lesions of the amygdala on both sides of the brain. In studies using the slides and emotional narrative used in experiments described above, Cahill and his colleagues[44] found that, unlike in normal subjects, the emotional narrative did not enhance long-term memory in two subjects who had amygdala lesions. The subjects' performance on the test for memory of the content of the slides was much like that of normal subjects given a beta blocker. These findings, as well as those of Elizabeth Phelps's studies of patients with amygdala lesions,[45] agree with the evidence from animal studies that the amygdala is critically involved in enabling emotional arousal to regulate memory consolidation. Interestingly, amnesic subjects who have damage to other brain regions have intact, though somewhat attenuated, enhanced memory for emotional material and, although the evidence is somewhat controversial, enhanced memory for emotionally arousing experiences appears to be relatively intact in early-stage Alzheimer's patients.[46]

The active amygdala

Additionally, and importantly, as discussed in chapter 3, the development of techniques, including PET (positron emission tomography) and fMRI (functional magnetic resonance imaging) for imaging human brain activity has enabled investigation of brain activity occurring during the encoding of long-term explicit memory. That is, it is now possible to 'peer into' the brain as learning is occurring, to see which brain regions are selectively active; but, as I noted in chapter 3, it is critical to ask specific questions when doing such peering. A study by Larry Cahill and his colleagues[47] was the first to try to determine, first, whether emotionally arousing material selectively influences amygdala activity assessed by brain (PET) imaging, and second, if it does, whether the degree of amygdala activity is related to subsequent long-term retention of the material. Adult male subjects first watched a brief series of portions of emotionally arousing (and unpleasant) or neutral films while their brains were scanned, using PET imaging (with radio-labelled glucose) to assess activation of various brain regions. Three weeks later they were given a surprise test of their memory for the films. Activity of the right amygdala induced by viewing of the emotionally arousing films correlated very highly (+0.93) with long-term memory of the films. When neutral films were viewed during PET imaging, amygdala activity did not correlate with remembrance of the films. It turned out to be important to note that all of the subjects in that study were males. A subsequent study[48] of amygdala activity and memory in adult female subjects obtained highly similar results. However, most interestingly, for females, activity of the *left* amygdala during the encoding of the emotionally arousing material correlated highly with subsequent retention. This intriguing sex difference in brain activity related to memory consolidation is yet another brain mystery that needs, and is getting, serious detective work.

Although it seems reasonable to conclude that emotional arousal was critical in creating the correlation between amygdala activity and subsequent memory, there are other possible interpretations. Perhaps it was the novelty or the unpleasantness of the films that caused the amygdala activity and influenced the subsequent memory of the films. Stephan Hamann and his colleagues[49] considered these alternative possibilities. Male subjects' brains were scanned, using PET (radio-labelled oxygen) while they viewed a series of pictures that were judged to be pleasant, unpleasant, interesting or novel, or neutral. Memory for both the pleasant and unpleasant pictures tested one month later correlated highly with amygdala activity assessed by PET. Interestingly, PET activity did not correlate with subsequent memory of the neutral or novel and interesting pictures.

In PET imaging studies, the effects are averaged over a series of stimulus events, such as brief films or pictures. The use of fMRI allows detection of alterations in brain activity induced by individual stimulus events in a series of events. John

Gabrieli and his colleagues[50] showed adult female subjects a series of pictures and gave them a surprise memory test three weeks later. The activity of the left amygdala induced by viewing each of the pictures correlated highly with the remembrance of the pictures: individual pictures that induced greater amygdala activity were better remembered. Moreover, the effect was greatest for pictures that were rated as the most emotionally arousing.

The findings of these brain imaging studies provide clear evidence that a little amygdala activity is good for creating lasting memory of events that initiated the activity – and that more amygdala activity is even better. All of these findings fit very well with the extensive evidence from animal studies of the role of the amygdala in modulating memory consolidation. The finding of Gabrieli and his colleagues that amygdala activity induced by each event in a series of events correlates with subsequent memory for each specific event provides additional evidence that amygdala activity is critical for modulating memory consolidation: stress hormones released by the adrenal gland clearly cannot differentially affect remembrance of individual events in a series of events. Stress hormones appear to help create lasting memories of events by influencing amygdala activity over a longer time scale, thus making stronger memories of series of experiences that, together, constitute an event or episode.

Those of us who have experienced a severe earthquake know that an earthquake can evoke strong emotional responses and strong memories. As briefly noted above, early-stage Alzheimer's patients generally retain the ability to create stronger memories of emotionally arousing experiences. Mori and his colleagues in Japan[51] studied the memories of thirty-six Alzheimer's patients who experienced the 1995 Kobe earthquake in their homes. That earthquake caused over 6000 deaths and widespread destruction of buildings, bridges and other structures. The subjects' memories were tested six weeks after the quake. The study also examined the volume of each subject's amygdala using MRI. In subjects with different degrees of brain atrophy and severity of cognitive impairment, the volume of the amygdala (average of left and right) correlated highly with the subjects' memory of their experiences at the time of the earthquake. Interestingly, the volume of the hippo-campal region did not. These findings provide yet more strong evidence that the amygdala is importantly involved in making emotional moments memorable.

Memory connections

Perhaps the most often asked, and certainly one of the most important, questions about memory is, 'What happens in the brain when memories are created?' The evidence discussed above very strongly and clearly indicates that amygdala activity plays a central role in creating memories of significant experi-ences; but the amygdala does not appear to be the place in the brain where the memories are made and maintained. Some neuroscientists, including Joe LeDoux[52] and Michael Davis,[53] have hypothesized that neural changes underlying the learning of cues associated with emotional responses such as fear occur within the amygdala, and have provided considerable evidence from animal studies that is consistent with that view. However, many studies, including some from my laboratory, have report-ed that complete lesions of the amygdala or lesions restricted to the basolateral amygdala do not prevent rats from learning and remembering fear-inducing experiences.[54] Additionally, as dis-cussed in some detail above, considerable evidence from research in my laboratory suggests that the amygdala influences long-term memory for emotionally significant events by regulat-ing the functioning of other brain regions involved in consolidat-ing lasting memory[55] – that is, your amygdala doesn't appear to be able to tell you where you were and what you were doing when you learned that Princess Diana had been killed in a car crash, or that planes had crashed into towers in New York City. The amygdala certainly made that memory possible – and strong; but the neural changes constituting your memory of that event are most likely located in circuits in other brain regions.

What are the 'building blocks' that create those circuits?
What are the neural 'units' of memory. Certainly, a complete
and detailed answer is not as yet available and is not likely to be
available soon; but research is continuing to reveal critical
clues about how brain cells and systems create and retain
memory.

An old and dominant hypothesis is that learning changes the
strength of connections between nerve cells and that the per-
sistence of the change creates lasting memory. Hebb's hypothesis discussed in chapter 3 is a variant of that general hypothesis.
Critical evidence relevant to it first appeared a quarter of a
century after Hebb's book appeared, and it is perhaps of particular significance that the evidence was based on studies of
changes in the activity of cells in the hippocampus – one of the
brain regions most often associated with the consolidation of
explicit memory. In their classical and seminal study,[56] using
rabbits as subjects, Tim Bliss and Terje Lomo placed an electrode in a neural path coming from the cortex into the hippocampus and another electrode in a region of the hippocampus
activated by the cortical pathway. Stimulation of the incoming
pathway produced a brief increase in activity of the hippocampal cells by activating existing synaptic connections
between the two groups of neurons. Repeated stimulation of
that incoming pathway induced a change in the connectivity
between the two groups of neurons by inducing changes in the
synapses connecting them.

This activity-dependent change in neuronal connectivity,
which Bliss and Lomo termed 'long-lasting potentiation' and
which is now referred to as 'long-term potentiation', or LTP, is
considered by perhaps most neuroscientists to reflect specific
changes in connections among neurons that may serve as a basis
for learning and memory. Because of that, research investigating
the nature and basis of LTP is one of the most intensive areas of
neuroscience. It is important to note that the view that LTP provides a basis for learning and memory is just that – a hypothesis;
but it is also important to note that the hypothesis is supported

by, or at least consistent with, evidence from many kinds of experiments. Drugs that block LTP generally impair learning and memory. For example, drugs that inhibit brain protein synthesis block the development of LTP as well as memory consolidation. Additionally, learning is often associated with the induction of LTP; and – of particular relevance to the issue of emotional arousal and lasting memory – there is extensive evidence that the basolateral amygdala regulates LTP induced in the hippocampus.[57] Thus, the findings of a large number of studies leave little doubt that, under many conditions, LTP is associated with learning; but what is missing, to date, is evidence that *critically* links LTP and learning[58] – evidence, that is, revealing whether or not LTP is *essential* for learning and memory and whether the LTP mechanisms are the substrate of time-dependent processes of memory consolidation.[59]

While that evidence is being intensely sought, the molecular and cellular mechanisms underlying the induction and maintenance of LTP are also being intensely, even 'feverishly', studied. If LTP reflects changes underlying the consolidation of memory, then understanding the molecular, biochemical and anatomical changes occurring at synapses mediating LTP will solve one of the greatest mysteries of memory.

It is not the *only* great mystery of memory, however: there are many. First, there are at least several forms of LTP. Each needs to be understood. Second, there are most likely other forms of neuroplasticity capable of providing a basis for memory. Third, making memory requires much more than creating connections between cells: inducing synaptic connections does not necessarily induce a memory. At the very least, memory is created by connecting some specific sets of neurons with other specific sets of neurons. These interconnected neurons must in some way or ways represent specific experiences; and the neurons must be parts of systems that deal with different kinds of information and are capable of generating appropriate responses. Memory may be based *on* but certainly involves much more *than* changes in synaptic connectivity.

As discussed earlier in this book, understanding the roles of different brain systems is one of the most important and challenging problems of memory. The role of the hippocampal system, in particular, is a complex puzzle. Most studies of LTP examine changes in the hippocampus of rats or mice, or in freshly prepared hippocampal brain slices that remain physiologically active for many hours when maintained in a dish containing appropriate solutions. Hippocampal LTP is studied for two major reasons. First, LTP was first discovered in hippocampal neurons. Thus, it should not be surprising that much subsequent research on LTP focused on the hippocampus. However, it should be noted that LTP has also been obtained in many other brain regions, including the amygdala (see reference 59); the hippocampus does not have an exclusive hold on LTP. A second major reason for studying LTP in the hippocampus, although obvious, is less well justified. Because of the extensive evidence suggesting that the hippocampal complex is critically involved in the consolidation of long-term explicit memory, it might seem appropriate to study LTP in that brain region; but it is clear that LTP occurring in the hippocampal region is not likely to provide *the* basis for long-term memory. After all, other brain regions are also involved in long-term memory and considerable evidence indicates that the hippocampal complex plays only a time-limited role in the consolidation of long-term explicit memory. Thus, the critical lasting changes must be located elsewhere in the brain. If LTP in the hippocampal complex plays a role in memory consolidation, the role might be either to hold information temporarily until it is transferred to other brain regions, such as the cerebral cortex, or to interact in some way with consolidation processes occurring in those other brain regions.[60] Whether the synaptic changes underlying LTP occur in those other brain regions when memory of memorable moments is being consolidated is another important mystery of memory that needs to be solved, and no doubt will be.

6 | Meandering and Monumental Memory

Many of us have played the game 'Chinese Whispers', or 'telephone', in which one person whispers a sentence into the ear of the neighbouring person in a circle and each person, in turn, whispers it to the next person. The sentence reported by the last person to receive the message typically bears little resemblance to the original sentence: it is usually ridiculously garbled. Why does this happen? In principle, there would be no reason to expect that the sentence should be distorted; but as each person listens to and remembers the sentence, the information is remembered and thus transmitted in at least a slightly different form. The greater the number of players in the game, the greater the opportunity for creating errors. This game is often considered as a model for the dispersion of rumours: as information is passed around, each person may 'remember' and, thus, transmit it in a slightly different way; remembering is usually, at least to some degree, creative *mis*-remembering. This is not news to wives – or to husbands – or to children listening to their parents remembering that a specific event happened in quite different ways.

Creative remembering

Remembering events is a creative act.[1] Although highly rehearsed material, such as the alphabet, favourite poems or songs and terms used frequently with your family and friends and associated with your hobbies, is accurately remembered and rarely forgotten, the ordinary events of daily life usually create fragile records. As discussed in the previous chapter, extraordinary events, particularly emotionally arousing events, tend to be well remembered; but as we noted, most of those memories usually fade, very gradually, over time. Only the most traumatic experiences resist forgetting.

Remembering events, whether ordinary or significant, is not simply a matter of locating the otherwise perfectly preserved memory stored at some place(s) in the brain and retrieving it intact. New experiences are, of course, related to previous experiences as well as to our general knowledge of the world (semantic information). The terms 'remembering', 'recollecting' and 'recalling' quite accurately reflect what we must do when we experience or discuss a particular memory. We must 're-member', 're-collect' and 're-construct' as we 're-call'; and, because of the massive interconnectedness of the records of our personal experiences and general knowledge, it is often, if not usually, quite difficult to retain and remember experiences with great accuracy. Our memories often meander.

The British psychologist Sir Frederic Bartlett was the first to give serious attention to this important issue in his highly influential (but often overlooked) book entitled, appropriately, *Remembering*, which was published in 1932.[2] We are all story tellers. In remembering events we usually construct stories. We remember some details and some sequences in the event as well as the overall experience; but in recalling the event we also make use of our general knowledge of such events. There are general sequences for events such as shopping trips, family dinners, religious ceremonies, weddings, funerals, trips to the movies, museums, and so forth. When we recall such events and tell others about them, we draw on our general knowledge about such events and our own previous experiences of them, as well as on our specific memories of a specific event; but the recollections are not always (if ever) clearly distinguished.

However, the general knowledge we have accumulated enables us to recall and relay coherent stories from often fragmented recollections.

As Bartlett's findings clearly indicated, we can also tell reasonably coherent stories even when we lack full understanding of events; but the coherence can be created at the expense of accuracy. A well-known example discussed in his book is that of British subjects' recollections of a North American folk tale called 'The War of the Ghosts'. Briefly, at the beginning of the story a group of men in a canoe ask a young native American from Egulac to accompany them on a trip up a river to make war on the people there. The story continues as follows:

And the warriors went on up the river to a town on the other side of Kalama. The people came down to the water, and they began to fight, and many were killed. But presently the young man heard one of the warriors say: 'Quick, let us go home; that Indian has been hit.' Now he thought: 'Oh they are ghosts.' He did not feel sick but they said he had been shot. So the canoes went back to Egulac, and the young man went ashore to his house, and made a fire. And he told everybody and said: 'Behold, I accompanied the ghosts, and we went to fight. Many of our fellows were killed, and many of those who attacked us were killed. They said I was hit, and I did not feel sick.' He told it all, and then he became quiet. When the sun rose he fell down. Something black came out of his mouth. His face became contorted. The people jumped up and cried. He was dead.[3]

The subjects each read the story twice and then attempted to reproduce it, in precise detail, first after fifteen minutes and then, repeatedly, at increasing intervals. In general, the story became significantly shortened; more modern words were used; the story became more coherent and the significance of the ghosts became distorted. One subject's effort to recall the story was made after a delay of two and a half years:

Some warriors went to wage a war against the ghosts. They fought all day and one of their number was wounded. They returned home in the evening bearing their sick comrade. As the day drew to a close he became rapidly worse and the villagers came around him. At sunset he sighed: something black came out of his mouth. He was dead.[4]

One might suggest that this version of the story is a reasonable reflection of the original story, but it is clear that the recollected story left out a great many details and distorted others. Imagine the significance of this report if it had been courtroom testimony under oath: 'So,' says the attorney, 'it is your testimony that this young man was killed by ghosts. Is that correct?' What might appear to be a small change in the story could well be a critical change under some circumstances. Bartlett's findings anticipated the critically important issue of the reliability of witnesses' courtroom testimony discussed below; but more generally the findings clearly revealed that we must acknowledge that remembering is a creative act that accesses and uses much more than, as well as much less than, the information originally stored.

In discussing the studies of flashbulb memory in the previous chapter, I reviewed evidence indicating that the subject's recollections were *generally* accurate and reliable over time. In the study of subjects' memory of when, where and how they found out about the O. J. Simpson trial verdict,[5] for example, fifty per cent of the subjects had no memory distortions or only minor distortions when tested thirty-two months after the event. It is at least equally important to note that over forty per cent of the subjects had major distortions in their memory of the event. However, it is also important to recall that subjects who reported that they were highly stressed by witnessing a shop owner shoot and kill a robber had recollections that were ninety-three per cent accurate within two days of the shooting and eighty-eight per cent accurate several months later. Thus, it is clear that not all memories are 'Bartlettized'. Highly emotionally significant experiences are less susceptible to the many influences of the reconstructive act of remembering. Some memories meander more, some less. The stronger the memory is originally, the less the meandering. Well-rehearsed information is less subject to memory distortion. I doubt that you ever *mis*-remember that 16 comes before 15; but you might from time to time *mis*-remember that S comes before Q or that Y comes before V in the alphabet (unless you first recite the alphabet to yourself). You are not likely to forget your own home address, phone number(s) or e-mail address, if they have remained constant and you have used them frequently.

Remembering misinformation

A relatively simple study originally conducted by the psychologist James Deese[6] and further developed by Henry Roediger and Kathleen McDermott[7] reveals that it is relatively easy to create inaccurate memories. In these experiments subjects were asked to read a list including words such as: 'thread', 'pin', 'sewing', 'sharp', 'point', 'prick', 'thimble'. They were then asked whether words in another list, which included 'needle', were on the original list. They were not. Most subjects, however, were highly confident that 'needle' was on the original list. Although this might seem trivial, imagine for a moment the significance of these findings if it were critical in a murder trial to know whether the suspect had mentioned 'needle'. A little false memory might have a very large consequence.

Much more elaborate false memories can also be created. Elizabeth Loftus and her colleagues[8] have managed to convince adult subjects that when they were children they had become lost while shopping with relatives. The story told the subjects was a complete fabrication created by the experimenters. One female subject was told this story:

> You, your mom, Tien and Tuan, all went to the Bremerton K-Mart. You must have been five years old at the time. Your mom gave each of you some money to get a blueberry ICEE. You ran ahead to get

into the line first, and somehow you lost your way in the store. Tien found you crying to an elderly Chinese woman. You three then went together to get an ICEE.[9]

The subject agreed that she had been lost and commented:

> I vaguely remember walking around...crying. I thought I was lost for ever. I went to the shoe department [and] the handkerchief place...I circled around the store it seemed 10 times. I just remember walking around and crying. I do not remember the Chinese woman or the ICEE (but it would have been raspberry ICEE...) part. I don't even remember being found...I just remember feeling that nobody was going to find me. I was destined to be lost at K-Mart for ever.[10]

Not all of Loftus's subjects were susceptible to mis-remembering the fictitious stories they were told. Only about one fourth of her subjects developed a false – or partially false – memory; and in comparison with memories of true events, the subjects' reports of their false memories were shorter and less clear. Quite different results were found with children given false information. In a series of studies, Stephen Ceci and his colleagues[11] showed individual pre-school children a set of cards, each depicting a different event, once a week for ten weeks. After the child picked a card, the interviewer would read it to the child and then ask if that event had ever happened to them, saying, for example, 'Think real hard, and tell me if this ever happened to you.' One card read: 'Got finger caught in a mousetrap and had to go to the hospital to get the trap off.' When the children were interviewed at the end of the ten weeks by a different adult, fifty-eight per cent of them gave false (i.e. fabricated) narratives to at least one of the fictitious events depicted on the cards and twenty-five per cent of the children produced false narratives to most of the suggested events. In discussing these findings, Ceci commented: 'What was so surprising was the elaborateness of the children's narratives. They were embellished; the children would provide an internally coherent account of the context in which their finger got caught in the mousetrap as well as the affect associated with the event.'[12] But again, it is important to note that many of the children (forty-two per cent) did *not* create false narratives. Memories, including those of young children, do not always meander.

However, as Elizabeth Loftus and Katherine Ketcham discuss in their book *The Myth of Repressed Memory*[13], the lives of families can sometimes be destroyed when they do. The book reviews the claims made by adult children that they recovered formerly long-repressed memories of having been sexually assaulted by their parents many years ago. In many, if not most, cases, the so-called recovery of such 'repressed' memories was deliberately and actively aided by psychotherapists. As there is no scientifically accepted evidence that strong emotional memories (or any memories, for that matter) can be 'repressed' and subsequently 'recovered', such claims are, at best, of very dubious validity. Moreover, the extensive evidence indicating that false memories can be created by suggestions provides a compelling explanation of the origin of the claims. It is, as the title of a chapter in the Loftus and Ketcham book suggests, 'The truth that never happened'. Memories may sometimes meander in very dangerous and unfortunate ways. In one of many such cases, a jury in Wisconsin awarded a family $850,000 after concluding that a psychiatrist had implanted false memories in a woman, leading her to believe that she was sexually abused by her father and that her parents were members of a cult that forced others to have sex with animals and witness babies being killed and eaten. After the verdict, the attorney for the family commented that there was no defence for this kind of therapy and that the jury's action was a message that it had to be stopped. Verdicts of this kind and cost may well do just that.

Although children's and adults' memories of events are sometimes, perhaps often, subject to deliberate or accidental misinformation, that is clearly not always the case. We do manage to remember many events quite accurately and reliably. If we were not able to maintain accurate and reliable memories, our lives would be chaotic. Imagine having to wonder which home was yours, which car, which child? That, of course, is the plight of individuals suffering from Alzheimer's disease and other diseases and disorders of memory. For most of us, most of the time, our mis-remembering is usually of minor consequence; and again, for most of us, the strong memories created by repetition or emotionally arousing experiences are the memories that are least susceptible to influences of either deliberate or accidental misinformation. I doubt that I could convince you that Tony Blair was the Prime Minister of France, that the Tower of London is located in New York, that your birthday is on 30 February, that Elvis Presley was a vaudeville juggler, or that Luciano Pavarotti is a British soccer player; and if you have had an intensely traumatic experience, such as a severe automobile accident, I seriously doubt that I could convince you that the accident did not occur, or that it occurred in Greenland. On the contrary, the problem might be that of dealing with the consequences of having an unforgettable traumatic memory.

A black hole in mental life

When I was seventeen years old, a drunk driver's car hit the car I was driving on the left front side and ripped off the bumper and door. I fell on to the highway and immediately noted that my favourite jacket was torn. I noted my injuries, which were not critical, shortly after. I certainly remember where I was and what I was doing when my car was smashed into, and I remember many other details: it was late at night; there was a rock retaining wall on the right side. The driver of the other car smashed into that wall and was critically injured; but I was fortunate. The accident left me with only minor injuries and a very strong (but certainly not perfect) memory of the event. Many who have serious accidents or who are mugged, or raped, or who witness a terrible event have very strong and intrusive memories as well as sometimes debilitating nightmares and anxiety. It is estimated that perhaps ten to fifteen per cent of those who have traumatic experiences have post-traumatic stress disorder (PTSD). Fortunately, in many cases the symptoms subside within a few months, but for some, the PTSD is a lifetime affliction.

The horrors of warfare are the source of many cases of PTSD. In the past century (and no doubt for many prior centuries), soldiers traumatized by their battle experiences were called, at best, 'shell-shocked' and, at worst, malingerers. PTSD is now recognized as a serious disorder caused by traumatic events that are not ordinarily experienced and that constitute a serious threat. Common symptoms include '...recurrent distressing recollections, dreams, and flashbacks of the traumatic event. One striking feature of PTSD is its timelessness. A PTSD sufferer may repeatedly experience a traumatic event with emotion so fresh each time that it is as if the event were recurring.'[14] Studies of PTSD patients '...serve to illustrate in exaggerated pathological form the potentially lasting effects of stressful life events on emotional memory. Indeed, in extreme instances, the memory of the traumatic event may become a "black hole" in the mental life of the PTSD patient, attracting all associations to it.'[15]

In an extensive series of studies, Roger Pitman and his colleagues studied the emotional responses of Vietnam veterans suffering from PTSD when they were reminded of their experiences in Vietnam and compared them with the responses of healthy combat veterans. They constructed scripts based on the veterans' personal experiences and recorded electrophysiological measures while the scripts were read to the subjects. The following is an example based on an experience of a Vietnam veteran with PTSD:

You have just received a signal for a hasty ambush. You sit in the elephant grass trying to figure out your field of fire. Then you hear them coming, talking and laughing and making jokes. You hold your breath, and your heart stops. You freeze, like you can't move.

Their voices keep on getting louder and louder. When they get right in front of you, you can see them from the waist down, with their AKs slung. You count them as they pass. When you get to four, all shit breaks loose. You pull your trigger and hold it down. The next thing you know, you're staring at a dead Gook's feet. Your teammates are yelling, 'Get up. We gotta go!' Now your heart is pounding, and you feel jittery all over, like you want to run, but there's no place to go. You stand up and see the top of the Gook's head blown off, his brains glaring in the sun. You've never seen blood and guts before. You feel sick to your stomach and in a state of shock.[16]

In comparison with healthy combat veterans, the veterans suffering from PTSD had greatly increased heart rate and blood pressure while listening to the narratives. Pitman and Orr noted the 'timelessness' of highly elevated physiological responses recorded from World War II veterans recalling traumatic experiences that had occurred many decades earlier. Although most memories fade over time, traumatic memories may last a lifetime.

A curious and no doubt significant feature of PTSD is that the disorder often has a delayed onset. Although the creation of the memory of the traumatic event is not delayed, the other symptoms may increase over time after the event. Pitman and Orr suggested that stress hormones may be responsible for the 'incubation' of PTSD: '...recall of the traumatic event may lead to re-releases of stress hormones that further enhance the strength of the memory trace, leading to a greater likelihood of its intruding again, with yet further releases of stress hormones. The result may be a positive feedback loop, in which subclinical PTSD may escalate into clinical PTSD.'[17] A clear implication of this hypothesis is that it should be possible to prevent, or at least decrease, the development of PTSD by blocking the actions of stress hormones released by the repeated remembrance of the traumatic experience.

As discussed extensively in the previous chapter, there is considerable evidence that the stress hormone epinephrine and the neurotransmitter norepinephrine play key roles in enhancing the consolidation of emotionally significant experiences; and there is also considerable evidence, from both animal and human studies, that beta blockers – that is, drugs that block ß-adrenergic receptors normally activated by epinephrine and norepinephrine – prevent the enhancing effects of emotional arousal on the consolidation of long-term memory. Such findings suggest that beta blockers given to individuals after they have experienced a traumatic experience may block the development of PTSD by preventing the enhancement of the memory of the trauma that would otherwise be induced by each recurrence of the memory. Several recent studies have provided evidence that is consistent with this hypothesis. In one study,[18] patients in an emergency department who had experienced a traumatic experience were administered the beta blocker propranolol or a placebo within six hours of the trauma and four times daily for ten days. The propranolol dose was then gradually decreased over nine subsequent days. One month after the trauma, the patients given propranolol had fewer symptoms of PTSD; two months later they had lower physiological responses, compared to those of the placebo-treated patients, when they were asked to 'image' the traumatic experience. In another study, using similar procedures,[19] propranolol given to patients within twenty hours after the traumatic experience significantly reduced the symptoms of PTSD assessed two months after the traumatic event. These studies, which were based *explicitly* on the findings of experimental studies of the effects of propranolol on emotionally influenced memory in animal and human subjects, provide strong evidence supporting the hypothesis that blocking the action of the stress hormone epinephrine may attenuate or even *prevent* the development of PTSD. It may not be possible to fill the 'black holes' in mental life created by PTSD, but these findings suggest that it may be possible to prevent the creation of such horrific holes. After all, although most of us might like to be able to remember better, there are many of us who would like to be better at forgetting.

Unforgettable

Shelves of bookshops are loaded with books filled with promises of techniques for improving memory. Shelves of healthfood stores are filled with packages of herbs with labels promising memory-boosting powers. The books and packages of herbs are not gathering dust: sales are booming. Sales of the herb ginkgo biloba in the US yield approximately a quarter of a billion dollars a year, despite very minimal evidence, at best, that it does anything other than help to increase the US Consumer Confidence Index. All of this evidence indicates that we want to have stronger, longer-lasting memories. We appear to want our experiences to be unforgettable; but should we want such memories? We should be very careful what we wish for. Certainly, as discussed above, there are many very specific experiences that we would very much like to be able to forget; and there is no need for us to remember every minor micro-detail of each of our daily experiences. The critical need is for *selective* memory of things that are important and useful. As the psychologist William James commented: 'Selection is the very keel on which our mental ship is built...If we remembered everything, we should, on most occasions be as ill off as if we remembered nothing. It would take as long for us to recall a space of time as it took the original time to elapse, and we should never get ahead with our thinking.'[20] Thus, in the long term, most of our trivial experiences are, and should be, forgettable. From this perspective it is most fortunate that the promises on the labels of packages of so-called memory-boosting herbs are unfulfilled. To consider in more detail why we may wish not to have the herbs fulfil our wishes, it is instructive to consider some cases of individuals who have extraordinary memories.

First, some fiction. In his short story 'Funes the Memorious',[21] the great Argentine author Jorge Luis Borges wrote about a young Uruguayan man who had been thrown from a horse and lay paralysed on a bed. When he was loaned several books, in Latin, including Pliny's *Naturalis historia*, he very quickly read them and discussed

> ...in Latin and in Spanish, the cases of prodigious memory recorded in the *Naturalis historia;* Cyrus, king of the Persians, who could call every soldier in his armies by name; Mithridates Eupator, who administered the law in the twenty-two languages of the empire; Simonides, inventor of the science of mnemonics; Metrodorus, who practiced the art of faithfully repeating what he had heard only once. In obvious good faith, [Funes] was amazed that such cases be considered amazing.

Funes said, 'I alone have more memories than all mankind has had since the world has been the world...My world is like a garbage heap.' Borges wrote,

> In fact, Funes remembered not only every leaf of every tree of every wood, but also every one of the times he had perceived or imagined it. [Funes was]...let us not forget, almost incapable of ideas of a general, Platonic sort...I suspect that he was not very capable of thought. To think is to forget differences, generalize, make abstractions. In the teeming world of Funes, there were only details...[22]

Unimportant, unforgettable details.

Next, some well-documented amazing memories. In 1968, the eminent Russian neuropsychologist A. R. Luria published his English version of *A Little Book about a Vast Memory: The Mind of a Mnemonist.*[23] The book reports his thirty-year study of a failed musician and journalist who became a professional memory expert, or mnemonist. When he was a journalist, his editor noted that S, as he is called in the book, never took notes but could repeat assignments precisely word for word. As he was curious about S's memory ability, the editor sent him to see Luria, who quickly discovered that S's memory was virtually unlimited in capacity and accuracy. Given a series of as many as seventy words or numbers, S could readily reproduce the series in order, or even in reverse order. In a typical experiment he was shown a table containing several columns of numbers. After examining the table of numbers for a few minutes he was able to recall them in columns, in reverse order, or in diagonals. You might try this yourself or ask a friend to try this feat of memory. Good luck! It should be a very good friend, one that is not likely to think that you are trying to make her/him look foolish. After intensive testing of S on sessions separated by days, weeks or years, Luria came to the conclusion that, the capacity of S's memory and the durability of his memory traces were unlimited. This remarkable memory ability enabled S to become a professional mnemonist.

Interestingly, his major problem as an entertainer was that his memory was *too* perfect. He frequently gave several performances each evening. In recalling numbers written on a blackboard and then concealed, he had great difficulty ignoring his memory of numbers written on the blackboard during earlier performances that evening, or even during performances on previous evenings. As Luria asked, 'How do we explain the tenacious hold these images had on his mind, his ability' to retain them not only for years but for decades? ... What explanation was there for the fact that ... S could select at will any series 10, 12 or even 17 years after he had originally memorized it? How had he come by this capacity for indelible memory traces?'[24] Perhaps it might help you or your friend to know that S perceived objects as having peculiar tastes, sounds and colours, a capacity termed 'synaesthesia', and that the synaesthesia aided his recollection. He commented: 'I recognize a word not only by the images it evokes but by a whole complex of feelings that image arouses. It's hard to express ... it's not a matter of vision or hearing but some over-all sense I get. Usually I experience a word's taste and weight...'[25]

Knowing that seems unlikely to help you when you try the memory feat above; but S's phenomenal memory was of little help to him in his normal daily life – on the contrary. His experiences, as those of Funes the Memorious, were complexly entangled with his memories. He wrote, 'The things I see when I read aren't real, they don't fit the context. If I'm reading the description of some palace, for some reason the main rooms always turn out to be those in the apartment I lived in as a child.' Throughout his life he changed jobs frequently and seemed to fail at all. Luria concluded, '... one would be hard put to say which was more real for him: the world of imagination in which he lived, or the world of reality in which he was but a temporary guest.'[26] S lived the life of the fictional Funes the Memorious – perhaps equally unsuccessfully.

Another mnemonist, V.P., was discovered by Earl Hunt and Tom Love at the University of Washington.[27] V.P. was born in Riga, Latvia, a city, very interestingly, close to the town where S spent his early years. He had schooling, as did S, that greatly emphasized memorization. It soon became clear that he had extraordinary memory capability. By the age of five he had memorized the street map of his city as well as the railway and bus timetables. When he was eight years old he began to play chess and chess became his major interest. V.P. finished college in the US and did some graduate work, but at the time he was studied he was working as a clerk in a store. As a chess expert, V.P. was reported to play up to seven simultaneous chess matches while blindfolded. He could play at least sixty corre-spondence games of chess without using written records. He performed well on an IQ test (136) and did particularly well on the memory subtests. He had a digit span (remembering just-presented strings of digits) of 21.5 compared to a digit span of less than eight for undergraduate subjects. His ability to recall columns and rows of numbers was comparable to that of S, but, unlike S, V.P. claimed that he did not use imagery. He did apparently use mnemonic aids, however. When recording a row of numbers he would regard them as a date and then ask himself what he was doing on that particular day. If you are still planning to try the test of memory of columns and rows of numbers on yourself or a friend, you can check to see if the use of dates makes the task easier. Again, good luck.

Early in this chapter, I presented a portion of the story of the 'War of the Ghosts' that Bartlett used in his studies of remembering. I also presented one subject's recollection of the tale obtained two and a half years after first recalling it. Without looking at either of these sections you might try to recall the 'War of the Ghosts' yourself – remember, the details are as important as the general story. If you do try to recall the story, write it down, and compare your version, as well as that of Bartlett's subject, with the recollection of V.P., obtained by Hunt and Love six weeks after reading the story:

The party went upriver to a point beyond Kalama, and when the people saw them approaching, they came down to the river, and they fought. In the heat of the battle, the young man heard somebody say: 'Quick let us go home. That Indian has been wounded.' They must be ghosts thought the young man, who felt no pain or injury. However, the party returned, and he walked from the river up to his village, where he lit a fire outside of his hut, and awaited the sunrise. 'We went with a war party to make war on the people upriver,' he told his people who had gathered around, 'and many were killed on both sides. I was told that I was injured but I feel alright. Maybe they were ghosts.' He told it all to the villagers. When the sun came up, a contortion came over his face. Something black came out of his mouth and he fell over. He was dead.[28]

If your recollection of the story is not quite as accurate as V.P.'s, you might read the original story again and try to remember it once again – or you might ask your friend to try to remember it. Why is it that some, obviously very rare, individuals have such an extraordinary ability to remember information? The simple answer is that we do not yet know. Nor do we as yet have any interesting specific hypotheses that might yield new insights. We do know that S and V.P. attended schools that required a great deal of memorizing, and they spent their early years in neighbouring cities in Latvia; but this information is not particularly useful in providing critical clues, as many children have had similar early experiences and there are, to our knowledge, not very many like S and V.P. Whether because of training or because of genetics, or perhaps some combination of the two, the brains of S and V.P., and others not yet studied who may be like them, differ from yours and mine; but at present the findings of such phenomenal memories provide no critical clues to their causes – only intriguing and highly important questions for future inquiry.

Most mysterious memory

I turn now to the most perplexing kinds of memory expressed by human subjects: the phenomenal memory ability sometimes seen in autistic children and adults. Approximately six per cent of autistic individuals have some exceptional abilities that are based, at least in part, on highly accurate memories. Their abilities go well beyond those of normal children and adults. Calendar calculation is one of the most commonly reported and studied abilities. I'll begin with a case of a young autistic man with an IQ of approximately 70 who was unable to learn to do relatively simple addition and subtraction but could give the day of the week for any day of the twentieth century.[29] Many calendar calculators can calculate days occurring over many centuries For example, one subject could give the weekday of any date from AD 1000 to 2000. Calendar calculation abilities in different individuals are reported to range from five years to 40,000 years.[30] One set of identical autistic twins were both able to do calendar calculations. One of the twins was especially successful in performing them. His range was at least 6000 years, which is well beyond that of any conventional perpetual calendar. Interestingly, his answers were incorrect for dates prior to 1582, the year that the Gregorian calendar replaced the Julian calendar.[31] Of course, anyone given the proper instructions can do calendar calculations, but it is not a simple task. Consider the following:

One method involves starting with the last two digits of the year involved, dividing these by four and adding the integer part to the dividend, ignoring the remainder. A number between 0 and 6, representing the indicated month, is then added and, finally the day of the month is added to the running total. This total is then divided by seven, the result ignored but the remainder noted. This remainder is then used to enter a table of days of the week to obtain the answer.[32]

If you or your friend that you asked to remember the 'War of the Ghosts' feel up to the challenge, you might simply use the instructions above and quickly find out the day of the week on which the first successful aeroplane flight occurred on 17 December 1903. It may take a while to do that. Autistic savants can determine that specific day within seconds, without the aid of a book, calendar calculator or computer. So, how do they do it? Despite intensive study of calendar calculators, no simple answers have been obtained and no simple hypotheses proposed. Clearly, much memory is required; but it is a different kind of memory from that which enables normal arithmetic calculations, and it is very different from the other kinds of memory revealed by individuals with low IQs.

What clues are there? Some autistic savants are known to have had access to perpetual calendars; but so did their parents, and the parents did not acquire the ability. You may wish to get a perpetual calendar, study it, and see if you can do calculations of the kinds summarized above. Again, good luck. The best hypothesis (i.e. guess, in this case) is that the ability is based on the extraordinary development of very specific implicit calculation strategies – that is, the savants appear to be able to deduce rules, learn, remember and apply them.[33] Of course, all of this is accomplished without any ability to explain why or how it is done; but how does anyone with extraordinary talent explain the origin of that talent? Non-autistic talented individuals can certainly talk about their talent, but the talk does not provide an explanation of its origin.

The ability to abstract is also revealed by other artistic

talents of some autistic savants. One such was reported to be able to play music in the style of several composers. It is also of considerable interest that autistic savants who are graphic artists require less information than do IQ-matched controls in order to identify incomplete pictures of objects. Such talents have resulted in some outstanding accomplishments. The crayola-drawn paintings of the legally blind autistic savant Richard Wawro sell for up to $10,000. Alonzo Clemons is an autistic savant who has what is described as an uncanny ability to create detailed animal figures out of clay, usually within an hour. His sculptures, which are displayed at the Driscol Galleries in Aspen, Colorado, reveal a remarkable knowledge of detail and exceptional talent as a sculptor. He is able to glance at a two-dimensional image of an animal and within a few minutes create a three-dimensional wax replica that is not only aesthetically exciting but anatomically accurate in minute detail. His best-known work is a life-sized sculpture of horses entitled *Three Frolicking Foals*. Such artistic talent requires, of course, exceptional memory – a very special kind of exceptional memory.

Remembrance: reflected and restrained

What enables the unique and exceptional talents of these autistic savants – individuals who have low IQs and limited abilities to care for themselves? Why don't you and I have these special talents? What are the essential differences between the brains of autistic savants and those of the rest of us? Understanding their brains could well provide critical insights into how all of us learn and remember. One obvious possibility is that the lack of development of some brain areas or processes may enable the excessive elaboration of other brain regions required for the expression of such unusual talents. Another more intriguing possibility is that all of us may have brains that could potentially allow such exceptional talents, but the normal functioning of our intact brains may prevent the expression of unusual talent.

The many systems of our brains constantly interact in enabling us to acquire, retain and use many kinds of information. Such interaction may inhibit the unique functioning of specific brain systems that would otherwise enable greater memory and creativity. Thus, perhaps all of our brains may have the capacity for monumental memories that enable very special talents; but that is a subject for yet another unwritten chapter, based on the workings of the memory systems of our brains yet to be investigated and understood. Another major mystery of memory – waiting to be solved.

7 | Memorabilia: Summing Up

Memorabilia are things worth remembering. So, in this brief summary, we will recall some things worth remembering about memory. In a little over a century since the beginning of the scientific study of memory much has been learned about the workings of memory and the brain processes that enable them. First, it was important to learn, despite centuries of scepticism, that memory can be studied objectively, using the general methods and techniques appropriate for any scientific inquiry. Next, it was essential to develop the specific methods required for investigating animal and human memory. It was also essential to discover the critical lessons provided by disorders of human memory. Finally, the development of many kinds of research techniques has enabled investigations of the brain systems and neurobiological machinery that coordinate and create fleeting or lasting representations of our experiences.

Even before the beginning of the scientific research, much was written about memory. William James[1] provided perhaps the best pre-scientific (that is, pre-experimental) thinking about memory. He distinguished between recent memory and lasting memory and considered habits as altogether different kinds of memory. His distinctions are honoured today in investigations of short-term memory, long-term memory and motor learning. We have learned that the brain also honours these distinctions. Different brain regions bear the primary responsibility for handling each form of memory as well as the orchestration of the interactions among them.

After the dawn of scientific research on learning and memory the pioneering giants, including Pavlov[2] and Thorndike,[3] created methods for studying memory in animals, and others, including especially Tolman,[4] revealed that much animal learning, like human learning, consists of learning about the predictability of our experiences. Each experience enables us to retain information that allows us to make highly reasonable predictions about the part of the world we live in, and use that information to behave, usually, appropriately.

We learned from Hebb's integrative and influential book[5] more about the distinction between short- and long-term memory as well as the suggested importance of post-learning neural reverberatory activity in creating structural changes required for lasting memory. At that same time in the mid-twentieth century the experimental findings of Duncan and others, indicating that treatments interfering with brain functioning administered shortly after learning impaired memory, reactivated interest in Müller and Pilzecker's[6] long-neglected memory consolidation hypothesis. These findings stimulated my own research,[7] as well as those of others, investigating the memory-enhancing effects of drugs and other treatments administered to animal and human subjects after learning. These studies led, in turn, to our discovery that stress hormones released by training or administered after training could also enhance memory consolidation. The studies also revealed that drugs and stress hormones influencing memory consolidation act via a specific brain region, the basolateral amygdala, which regulates memory consolidation through its influences on different forms of memory processed by different brain regions.[8]

Clinical observations as well as observational and experimental studies have provided considerable evidence that emotionally arousing experiences tend to be well remembered. Although we all know that, or think we do, it is important that this conclusion is well documented by extensive evidence. The evidence that stress-released hormones and activation of the amygdala can produce strong memories in animal and human subjects seems to provide an explanation for these well-documented effects. It is also now reasonably well known that especially traumatic experiences can produce intense, long-lasting traumatic memories, or post-traumatic stress disorder. Pitman[9] has suggested that stress-released hormones may also play a critical role in the development of PTSD. The evidence suggesting that the development of PTSD is blocked or attenuated by treating subjects with a drug that blocks the actions of the stress hormone epinephrine provides compelling support for this hypothesis.

Our memories are not perfect. Bartlett's early findings[10] and Loftus's more recent studies[11] have shown that weak memories are easily influenced and that, under some circumstances, completely false 'memories' can be created. Loftus's findings have highly important implications for understanding the reliability, or otherwise, of eyewitness testimony. In contrast, strong memories, whether due to extensive rehearsal or intensive emotional arousal, are resistant to forgetting.

Those of us who may wish for stronger memories should consider the consequences of having exceptional memory ability. Borges's fictional narrative of the sad plight of Funes the Memorious,[12] whose memory was 'like a garbage heap' – a large pile of unsorted minutiae – closely paralleled Luria's[13] account of S, the remarkable mnemonist who had a remarkably unsatisfactory life. Excessively strong memories apparently come at a very high personal price. The remarkable talents of autistic savants who can calculate calendars, paint glorious pictures or sculpt amazing animal figures are matched by their lack of other forms of memory abilities and their inability to lead normal lives.

These are a few of the memorabilia discussed in this book. There are many other aspects and facts of memory and its neural bases that I have not discussed. I have provided references to other excellent books dealing with other aspects of memory, including its cellular mechanisms.[14]

Our lives require that we record our experiences. As I noted at the beginning of this book, we can't go onstage – or anywhere, for that matter – without memory. It is essential that we preserve records of our experiences. It is fortunate that our brains do this for us – efficiently and effectively, most of the time; and in a little over a century we have learned much about how our brains do this. There is much, much more remaining to be discovered, however. Memories, as we have seen, are complex. Our brains are extraordinarily complex. New discoveries will require new hypotheses and, most likely, new techniques and methods. The final chapters providing a complete and detailed explanation of what our brains do to preserve the presence of the past are not likely to be written any time soon.

Notes and References

Chapter 1: The Mystery of Memory

1. The evidence concerning different forms of memory as well as the neurobiological bases is presented in several recent books: Schacter, Daniel L., *The Seven Sins of Memory*, Houghton Mifflin Company, Boston, 2001; Eichenbaum, H., and Cohen, N. J., *From Conditioning to Conscious Recollection: Memory Systems of the Brain*, Oxford University Press, New York, 2001, 2002; Bourtchouladze, R., *Memories Are Made of This*, Weidenfeld and Nicolson, London, 2002; Squire, Larry R. and Kandel, E. R., *Memory From Mind to Molecules*, Scientific American Library, New York, 1999; Dudai, Y., *Memory from A to Z*, Oxford University Press, Oxford, 2002.
2. Ebbinghaus, H., *Über das Gedächtnis*, Drucker and Humblat, Leipzig, 1885.
3. *LA Times*, 2 February 2000.

Chapter 2: Dogs, Cats, Chimps and Rats: Habits and Memory

1. James, W., *Principles of Psychology*, Henry Holt and Company, New York, 1890, pp. 104, 115.
2. Tulving, Endel, *Elements of Episodic Memory*, Oxford University Press, New York, 1983.
3. James, W., pp. 104–15.
4. Pavlov, I. P., *Conditioned Reflexes*, Oxford University Press, London, 1927.
5. Thorndike, E. L., 'Animal intelligence: an experimental study of the associative processes in animals' *Psychological Review*, Monograph Supplement 2, no. 8 (1898).
6. Pavlov, I. P., *Experimental Psychology and Other Essays*, Philosophical Library, New York, 1957, pp. 43–4.

7. Pavlov, I. P., (1927), pp. 147–8.

8. Watson, J. B., 'Psychology as the behaviorist views it', *Psychological Review*, 20 (1913), pp. 158–77.

9. Tolman, E. C., *Purposive Behavior in Animals and Men*, The Century Co., New York, 1932.

10. Hull, C. L., *Principles of Behavior*, Appleton-Century-Crofts, New York, 1943.

11. Hull, C. L. (1943), p. v.

12. Hull, C. L. (1943), p. 27.

13. Köhler, W., *The Mentality of Apes*, Harcourt, Brace, 1925.

14. Lashley, K. S. and McCarthy, D. A. 'The survival of the maze habit after cerebellar injuries', *Journal of Comparative Psychology* 6 (1926), 423–33.

15. Lorenz, K., 'Innate bases of learning', in Pribram, K., *On the Biology of Learning*, Harcourt, Brace and World, New York, (1969), p. 47.

16. Liddell, H. S., 'The conditioned reflex', in Moss, F. A. (ed.), *Comparative Psychology*, Prentice-Hall, Englewood Cliffs, NJ, 1942.

17. Tolman, E. C. (1932), p. 8.

18. Hull, C. L. (1943), p. 27.

19 Rescorla, R., 'Pavlovian Conditioning. It's not what you think it is', *American Psychologist* 43 (1988), 151–60.

20. Davis, M. and Schlesinger, L. S., 'Temporal specificity of fear conditioning: effects of different conditioned stimulus-unconditioned stimulus intervals on the fear-potentiated startle effect', *Journal of Experimental Psychology, Animal Behavior Processes* 15 (1989), 295–310.

21. Thompson R. F., and Krupa D. J., 'Organization of memory traces in the Mammalian brain', *Annual Review of Neuroscience* 17 (1994), 519–49.

22. Lawrence, D. H., and di Rivera, J., 'Evidence for relational transposition', *The Journal of Comparative and Physiological Psychology* 47 (1954), 465–71.

23. Bunsey, S., and Eichenbaum, H., 'Conservation of hippocampal memory function in rats and humans', *Nature* 379 (1966), 255–7.

24. Tolman, E. C., 'There is more than one kind of learning', *Psychological Review* 56 (1949), 144–55.

25. Scoville, W. B. and Milner, B., 'Loss of recent memory after bilateral hippocampal lesions', *Journal of Neurological Neurosurgery and Psychiatry* 20 (1957), 11–21.

26. Fortin, N. J., Agster, K. L. and Eichenbaum, H. B., 'Critical role of the hippocampus in memory for sequences of events', *Nature Neuroscience* 5 (2002), 458–62.

27. Packard, M. G. and McGaugh, J. L., 'Inactivation of hippocampus or caudate nucleus with lidocaine differentially affects expression of place and response learning', *Neurobiology of Learning and Memory* 65 (1996), 65–72.

28. Garcia, J., and Koelling, R. A., 'Relation of cue to consequence in avoidance conditioning', *Psychonomic Science* 4 (1966), 123–4.

Chapter 3: The Short and Long of It

1. James, W. (1890), p. 643.

2. Ribot, T., *Diseases of Memory*, Appleton, New York, 1882.

3. Whitty, C. W. M. and Zangwill, O. L., 'Traumatic amnesia', in Whitty and Zangwill (eds.), *Amnesia*, Appleton-Century-Crofts, 1966, pp. 92–108.

4. Russell, W. R. and Nathan, P. W., 'Traumatic amnesia', *Brain* 69 (1946), 280–300.

5. Müller, G. E., and Pilzecker, A., 'Experimentalle beitrage zur lehre vom gedächtnis', *Z. Psychol.* 1, (1900), 1–288.

6. Burnham, W. H., 'Retroactive Amnesia: Illustrative cases and a tentative explanation', *American Journal of Psychology* 14 (1903), 382–96.

7. Cerletti, U. and Bini, L., 'Electric shock treatment', *Boll. Accad. Med. Roma* 64 (1938), 36.

8. Duncan, C. P., 'The retroactive effect of electroshock on learning', *Journal of Comparative and Physiological Psychology* 42 (1949), 32–44.

9. McGaugh, J. L., and Herz, M. J., *Memory Consolidation*, Albion Publishing Company, San Francisco, 1972, p. 204; McGaugh, J. L., 'Time-dependent processes in memory storage', *Science* 153 (1966), 1351–58; McGaugh, J. L., 'Memory: a century of consolidation', *Science* 287 (2000), 248–51.

10. Hebb, D. O., *The Organization of Behavior*, Wiley, New York, 1949.

11. Hebb, D. O. (1949), p. 62.

12. Agranoff, B. W., Davis, R. E. and Brink, J. J., 'Memory fixation in the goldfish', *Proceedings, National Academy of Sciences, USA* 54 (1965, 788–93.

13. Izquierdo, I., Barros, D. M., Mello e Souza, T., de Souza, M. M. and Izquierdo, L. A., 'Mechanisms for memory types differ', *Nature* 393 (1998), 635–6.

14. Karni A., Sagi D., 'The time course of learning a visual skill', *Nature* 365 (1993), 250–52.

15. Shadmehr, R. and Holcomb, H. H., 'Neural correlates of motor memory consolidation', *Science* 277 (1997), 821–5.

16. Weinberger, N. M., 'Tuning the brain by learning and by stimulation of the nucleus basalis', *Trends in Cognitive Sciences* 2 (1998), 271–3.

17. Galvan, V. V. and Weinberger, N. M., 'Long-term consolidation and retention of learning-induced tuning plasticity in the auditory cortex of the guinea pig', *Neurobiology of Learning and Memory* 77 (2002), 78–108.

18. Rose, S. P. R., 'Time-dependent processes in memory formation revisited', in Gold, P. E. and Greenough, W. T. (eds.), *Memory Consolidation: Essays in Honor of James L. McGaugh*, American Psychological Association, Washington, DC, 2001, pp. 113–28; Menzel, R. and Müller, U., 'Learning and memory in honeybees: from behavior to neural substrates', *Annual Review of Neuroscience* 19 (1996), 379–404; Emptage, N. J., and Carew, T. J., 'Long-term synaptic facilitation in the absence of short-term facilitation in Aplysia neurons', *Science* 262 (1993), 253–6.

19. Barbizet, J., 'Defect of memorizing of hippocampal-mammillary origin: a review', *Journal of Neurology and Neurosurgery Psychology* 26 (1963), 127–35.

20. Scoville, W. B. and Milner, B. (1957).

21. Milner, B., 'Amnesia following operation on the temporal lobes', in Whitty, C. W. M. and Zangwill, O. L. (eds.), *Amnesia*, Appleton-Century-Crofts, 1966, pp. 109–33.

22. Corkin, S., 'What's new with the amnesic patient H.M.?', *Nature Reviews Neuroscience* 3 (2002), 153–60.

23. Teng, E. and Squire, L. R., 'Memory for places learned long ago is intact after hippocampal damage', *Nature* 400 (1999), 675–7.

24. Warrington, E. K., and Weiskrantz, L., 'The effect of prior learning on subsequent retention in amnesic patients', *Neuropsychologia* 12 (1974), 419–28.

25. Squire, L. R., Cohen, N. J. and Zouzounis, J. A. 'Preserved memory in retrograde amnesia: sparing of a recently acquired skill', *Neuropsychologia* 22 (1984), 145–52; Graf, P., Squire, L. R. and Mandler, G. 'The information that amnesics do not forget', *Journal of Experimental Psychology* 10 (1984), 164–78.

26. Whitty, C. W. M. and Zangwill, O. L. (1966), p. 106.

27. Brown, A. S., 'Consolidation theory and retrograde amnesia in humans', *Psychonomic Bulletin and Review* 9 (2002), 403–25.

28. Squire, L. R. and Alvarez, P., 'Retrograde amnesia and memory consolidation: a neurobiological perspective', *Current Opinion in Neurobiology* 5 (1995), 169–77.

29. Squire, L. R., Slater, P. C., and Chace, P. M., 'Retrograde amnesia: temporal gradient in very long-term memory following electroconvulsive therapy', *Science* 187 (1975), 77–9.

30. Kim, J. J., and Fanselow, M. S., 'Modality-specific retrograde amnesia of fear', *Science* 256 (1992), 675–7.

31. Rugg, M. D., 'Memories are made of this', *Science* 218 (1998), 1151–2.

32. Alkire, M. T., Haier, R. J., Fallon, J. H., and Cahill, L., 'Hippocampal, but not amygdala activity at encoding correlates with long-term, free recall of nonemotional material', *Proceedings, National Academy of Sciences, USA* 95 (1998), 14506–10.

33. Highly similar findings were obtained in other experiments using fMRI brain imaging: Brewer, J. B., Zhao, Z., Desmond, J. E., Glover, G. H., and Gabrieli, J. D. 'Making memories: brain activity that predicts how well visual experience will be remembered', *Science* 281 (1998), 1185–7; Wagner, A. D., Schacter, D. L., Rotte, M., Koutstaal, W., Maril, A., Dale, A. M., Rosen, B. R. and Buckner, R. L., 'Building memories: remembering and forgetting of verbal experiences as predicted by brain activity', *Science* 281 (1998), 1188–91.

34. Haist, F., Gore, J. B., and Mao, H., 'Consolidation of human memory over decades revealed by functional magnetic resonance imaging', *Nature Neuroscience* 4 (2001), 1139–45.

35. Maguire, E. A., Gadian, D. G., Johnsrude, I. S., Good, C. D., Ashburner, J., Frackowiak, R. S. J., and Frith, C. D., 'Navigation-related structural change in the hippocampi of taxi drivers', *Proceedings, National Academy of Sciences, USA* 97 (2000), 4398–403; Maguire E. A., Frackowiak, R. S. J. and Frith, C. D., 'Recalling routes around London: activation of the right hippocampus in taxi drivers', *Journal of Neuroscience* 17 (1997), 7103–10.

Chapter 4: Coaxing Consolidation: Making Memories Linger

1. Lashley, K. S., 'The effects of strychnine and caffeine upon the rate of learning', *Psychobiology I* (1917), 141–70.

2. McGaugh, J. L., and Petrinovich, L., 'The effect of strychnine sulphate on maze-learning', *The American Journal of Psychology* 72 (1959), 99–102.

3. Tolman, E. C. (1932).

4. McGaugh, J. L., 'Some neurochemical factors in learning', unpublished PhD thesis (1959), University of California, Berkeley.

5. McGaugh J. L., 'Involvement of hormonal and neuromodulatory systems in the regulation of memory storage', *Annual Review of Neuroscience* 12 (1989), 255–87; McGaugh, J. L., 'Dissociating learning and performance: drug and hormone enhancement of memory storage', *Brain Research Bulletin* 23 (1989), 339–45.

6. Petrinovich, L., Bradford, D. and McGaugh, J. L., 'Drug facilitation of memory in rats', *Psychonomic Science* 2 (1965), 191–2.

7. Fanselow, M. S., 'Factors governing one-trial contextual conditioning', *Animal Learning and Behavior* 18 (1990), 264–70; Kim, J. J., and Fanselow, M. S. (1992).

8. Inhibitory avoidance was originally studied by Bradford Hudson, a graduate student in E. D. Tolman's laboratory. Murray Jarvik modified the procedures for use in studies of retrograde amnesia for one-trial learning.

9. Castellano, C., and McGaugh, J. L., 'Retention enhancement with posttraining picrotoxin: lack of state dependency', *Behavioral and Neural Biology* 51 (1989), 165–70.

10. Rose, S. P. R. (2001).

11. McGaugh, J. L., 'Drug facilitation of learning and memory', *Annual Review of Pharmacology* 13 (1973), 229–41; McGaugh, J. L., and Herz, M. J., *Memory Consolidation*, Albion Publishing Company, San Francisco, 1972. Drugs can also enhance the extinction of fear-based memory in rats if they are administered shortly before or after extinction training in which a cue previously associated with a foot-shock is no longer followed by the footshock. See McGaugh, J. L., Castellano, C. and Brioni, J. D. 'Picrotoxin enhances latent extinction of conditioned fear', *Behavioral Neuroscience*, 104 (1990), 262–65; Walker, D L., Ressler, K. J., Lu, K. T. and Davis, M., 'Facilitation of conditioned fear extinction by systematic administration or intra-amygdala infusions of d-cycloserine as assessed with fear-potentiated startle in rats', *Journal of Neuroscience*, 22 (2002), 2343–51.

12. Tomaz, C., Dickinson-Anson, H. and McGaugh, J. L., 'Basolateral amygdala lesions block diazepam-induced anterograde amnesia in an innhibitory avoidance task', *Proceedings, National Academy of Sciences, USA* 89 (1992), 3615–19.

13. Da Cunha, C., Wolfman, C., Huang, C., Walz, R., Koya, R., Bianchin, M., Medina, J. H. and Izquierdo, I., 'Effect of posttraining injections of flumazenil into the amygdala, hippocampus and septum on retention of habituation and of inhibitory avoidance in rats', *Brazilian Journal of Medical and Biological Research* 24 (1991), 301–6.

14. Stratton, L. O. and Petrinovich, L., 'Posttrial injections of an anti-cholinesterase drug on maze learning in two strains of rats', *Psychopharmacologia* 5 (1963), 47–54. This is the first study reporting that memory is enhanced by modulating acetylcholine activity.

15. McGaugh, J. L. and Cahill, L., 'Interaction of neuromodulatory systems in regulating memory storage', *Behavioural Brain Research* 83 (1997), 31–8.

16. Goddard, G., 'Amygdaloid stimulation and learning in the rat', *Journal of Comparative and Physiological Psychology* 58 (1964), 23–30. McGaugh, J. L., and Gold, P. E., 'Modulation of memory by electrical stimulation of the brain', in Rosenzweig, M. R., and Bennett, E. L. (eds.), *Neural Mechanisms of Learning and Memory*, The MIT Press, 1976, pp. 549–60.

17. Gallagher, M., Kapp, B. S., Pascoe, J. P., and Rapp, P. R., 'A neuropharmacology of amygdaloid systems which contribute to learning and memory', in Ben-Air, Y. (ed.), *The Amygdaloid Complex*, Amsterdam, Elsevier/N. Holland, 1981, pp. 343–54.

18. McGaugh, J. L., Ferry, B., Vazdarjanova, A. and Roozendaal, B., 'Amygdala: Role in modulation of memory storage', in Aggleton, J. P. (ed.), *The Amygdala: A Functional Analysis*, Oxford University Press, London, 2000, pp. 391–423.

19. Quirarte, G. L., Galvez, R., Roozendaal, B. and McGaugh, J. L., 'Norepinephrine release in the amygdala in response to footshock and opioid peptidergic drugs', *Brain Research* 808 (1998), 134–40; Hatfield, T., Spanis, C. and McGaugh, J. L., 'Response of amygdalar norepinephrine to footshock and GABAergic drugs using *in vivo* microdialysis and HPLC', *Brain Research* 835 (1999), 340–45. McIntyre, C. K., Hatfield, T. and McGaugh, J. L., 'Amygdala norepinephrine levels after training produce inhibitory avoidance retention performance in rats', *European Journal of Neuroscience* 16 (2002), 1223–26.

20. Morris, R. G. M., 'Development of a water-maze procedure for studying spatial learning in the rat, *Journal of Neuroscience Methods* 11 (1984), 47–60.

21. White, N. M., and McDonald, R. J., 'Multiple parallel memory systems in the brain of the rat', *Neurobiology of Learning and Memory* 77 (2002), 125–84.

22. Packard, M. G., Cahill, L. and McGaugh, J. L., 'Amygdala modulation of hippocampal-dependent and caudate nucleus-dependent memory processes', *Proceedings, National Academy of Sciences, USA* 91 (1994), 8477–81; Packard, M. G., and Teather, L., 'Amygdala modulation of multiple memory systems: Hippocampus and caudate-putamen', *Neurobiology of Learning and Memory* 69 (1998), 163–203.

23. Packard, M. G., 'Glutamate infused post-training into the hippocampus or caudate-putamen differentially strengthens place and response learning', *Proceedings, National Academy of Sciences, USA* 96 (1999), 12881–6.

24. Young, M. P., 'The organization of neural systems on the primate cerebral cortex', *Proceedings, Royal Society of London B. Biological Sciences* 252 (1993), 13–18.

25. Packard, M. G., Introini-Collison, I. and McGaugh, J. L., 'Stria terminalis lesions attenuate memory enhancement produced by intracaudate nucleus injections of oxotremorine', *Neurobiology of Learning and Memory* 65 (1996), 278–82.

26. McGaugh, J. L., 'Memory consolidation and the amygdala: A systems perspective', *Trends in Neurosciences* 25 (2002), 456–61.

27. Izquierdo, I., Quillfeldt, J. A., Zanatta, M. S., Quevedo, J., Schaeffer, E., Schmitz, P. K. and Medina J. H., 'Sequential role of hippocampus and amygdala, entorhinal cortex and parietal cortex in formation and retrieval of memory for inhibitory avoidance in rats', *European Journal of Neuroscience* 9 (1997), 786–93.

28. Jenkins, J. G., and Dallenbach, K. M., 'Oblivescence during sleep and waking', *American Journal of Psychology* 35 (1924), 605–12.

29. Heine, R., 'Uber Wiedererkennen und ruckinirkinde Hemmung', *Z. Psychol.* 68 (1914), 161–236.

30. Fishbein, W., McGaugh, J. L., and Swarz, J. R., 'Retrograde amnesia: Electroconvulsive shock effects after termination of rapid eye movement sleep deprivation', *Science* 172 (1971), 80–82.

31. Bloch, V., Hennevin, E., and LeConte, P., 'Interaction between posttrial reticular stimulation and subsequent paradoxical sleep in memory consolidation processes', in Drucker-Colin, R. R. and McGaugh, J. L. (eds.), *Neurobiology of Sleep and Memory*, Academic Press, 1977, pp. 255–72.

32. Stickgold, R., James, L., and Hobson, J. A., 'Visual discrimination learning requires sleep after training', *Nature Neuroscience* 3 (2000), 1237–8.

33. Fischer, S., Hallschmid, M., Elsner, A. L., and Born, J., 'Sleep forms memory for finger skills', *Proceedings, National Academy of Sciences, USA* 99 (2002), 11987–91.

34. Wilson, M. A., and McNaughton, B. L., 'Reactivation of hippocampal ensemble memories during sleep', *Science* 265 (1994), 676–8.

35. Paré, D., 'Mechanisms of Pavlovian fear conditioning: has the engram been located?', *Trends in Neuroscience* 25 (2002), 436–7.

36. Gerard, R. W., 'The fixation of experience', in Delafresnaye, J. F. (ed.), *Brain Mechanisms and Learning*, Charles C. Thomas, 1961, pp. 21–35.

Chapter 5: Memorable Moments

1. Stratton, G. M., 'Retroactive hypermnesia and other emotional effects on memory', *Psychological Review* 26 (1919), 474–86.
2. Wagenaar, W. A., and Groeneweg, J., 'The memory of concentration camp survivors', *Applied Cognitive Psychology* 4 (1990), 77–87.
3. Brown, R., and Kulik, J., 'Flashbulb memories', *Cognition* 5 (1977), 73–99.
4. Conway, M., *Flashbulb Memories*, Lawrence Erlbaum Associates, Hove, UK, 1995.
5. Neisser, U., 'Snapshots or benchmarks', in Neisser, U. (ed.), *Memory Observed: Remembering in Natural Contexts*, W. H. Freeman, San Francisco, 1982, pp. 43–8, quoted from p. 45.
6. Thompson, C. P. and Cowan, T., 'Flashbulb memories: A nicer interpretation of a Neisser recollection', *Cognition*, 22, 199–200.
7. Bohannon, J. N., 'Flashbulb memories for the space shuttle disaster: A tale of two theories', *Cognition* 29 (1988), 179–96.
8. Neisser, U., Winograd, E., Bergman, E. T., Schreiber, C. A., Palmer, S. E. and Weldon, M. S., 'Remembering the earthquake: direct experience vs. hearing the news', *Memory* 4 (1996), 337–57.
9. Conway, M. A., Anderson, S. J., Larsen, S. F., Donnelly, C. M., McDaniel, M. A., McClelland, A. G. R., Rawles, R. E., and Logie, R. H., 'The formation of flashbulb memories', *Memory and Cognition* 22 (1994), 326–43.
10. Bohannon, J. N., 'Recall of the Hillsborough disaster over time: Systematic bases of 'flashbulb' memories', *Applied Cognitive Psychology*, 7, (1988) 129–38.
11. Schmolck, H., Buffalo, E. A. and Squire, L. R., 'Memory distortions develop over time: recollections of the O. J. Simpson trial verdict after 15 and 32 months', *Psychological Science* 22 (2000), 39–45.
12. Yuille, J. C., and Cutshall, J. L., 'A case study of eyewitness memory of a crime', *Journal of Applied Psychology* 71 (1986), 291–301.
13. Kleinsmith, L. J. and Kaplan, S., 'Paired associate learning as a function of arousal and interpolated interval', *Journal of Experimental Psychology* 65 (1963), 190–93.
14. Cahill, L. and McGaugh, J. L., 'A novel demonstration of enhanced memory associated with emotional arousal', *Consciousness and Cognition* 4 (1995), 410–21.
15. Heuer, F., and Reisberg, D., 'Vivid memories of emotional events: The accuracy of remembered minutiae', *Memory and Cognition* 18 (1990), 496–506.
16. Heuer, F. and Reisberg, D., 'Emotion, arousal and memory for detail', in Christianson, S-A (ed.), *The Handbook of Emotion and Memory:*

Research and Theory, Lawrence Erlbaum Associates, Hillsdale, 1992, pp. 151–80, quoted from p. 176.

17. Guy, S. and Cahill, L., 'The role of overt rehearsal in enhanced conscious memory for emotional events', *Consciousness and Cognition* 8 (1999), 114–22.

18. Stratton, G. M., 'Retroactive hypermnesia and other emotional effects on memory', *Psychological Review* 26 (1919), 474–86, quoted from p. 483.

19. Livingston, R. B., 'Reinforcement', in Quarton, G. C., Melnechuk, T., and Schmitt, F. O. (eds.), *The Neurosciences: A Study Program*, Rockefeller University Press, New York, 1967, pp. 514–76.

20. Kety, S. S., 'The biogenic amines in the central nervous system: Their possible roles in arousal, emotion and learning', in Schmitt, F. O. (ed.), *The Neurosciences*, Rockefeller University Press, 1970, quoted from p. 330.

21. McGaugh, J. L., and Herz, M. J. (1972).

22. Gerard, R. W., 'The fixation of experience', in Delafresnaye, J. F. (ed.), *Brain Mechanisms and Learning*, Charles C. Thomas, 1961, pp. 21–35, quoted from pp. 29–30.

23. Gold, P. E., and Van Buskirk, R., 'Facilitation of time-dependent memory processes with posttrial epinephrine injections', *Behavioral Biology* 13 (1975), 145–53.

24. Gold, P. E., and Van Buskirk, R., 'Posttraining brain norepinephrine concentrations: Correlation with retention performance of avoidance training and with peripheral epinephrine modulation of memory processing', *Behavioral Biology* 25 (1978), 509–20.

25. Introini-Collison, I., Saghafi, D., Novack, G. and McGaugh, J. L., 'Memory-enhancing effects of posttraining dipivefrin and epinephrine. Involvement of peripheral and central adrenergic receptors', *Behavioral Biology* 25 (1978), 509–20.

26. Gold, P. E., 'An integrated memory regulation system: From blood to brain', in Frederickson, R. C. A., McGaugh, J. L. and Felten, D. L., *Peripheral Signaling of the Brain: Role in Neural-immune Interactions, Learning and Memory*, Hogrefe & Huber, Toronto, 1991, pp. 391–419.

27. Williams, C. L., 'Contribution of brainstem structures in modulating memory storage processes', in Gold, P. E., and Greenough, W. T. (eds.), *Memory Consolidation: Essays in Honor of James L. McGaugh*, American Psychological Association, 2001, pp. 141–63.

28. Liang, K. C., Juler, R. G. and McGaugh, J. L., 'Modulating effects of post-training epinephrine on memory: involvement of the amygdala noradrenergic system', *Brain Research* 368 (1986), 125–33.

29. Gallagher, M., Kapp, B. S., Pascoe, J. P. and Rapp, P. R., 'A neuropharmacology of amygdaloid systems which contribute to learning and memory', in Ben-Air, Y. (ed.), *The Amygdaloid Complex*, Amsterdam, Elsevier/N. Holland, 1981, pp. 343–54.

30. Hatfield, T. and McGaugh, J. L., 'Norepinephrine infused into the basolateral amygdala posttraining enhances retention in a spatial water maze task', *Neurobiology of Learning and Memory* 71 (1999), 232–9; Ferry, B. and McGaugh, J. L., 'Clenbuterol administration into the basolateral amygdala post-training enhances retention in an inhibitory avoidance task', *Neurobiology of Learning and Memory* 72 (1999), 8–12.

31. Liang, K. C. and McGaugh, J. L., 'Lesions of the stria terminalis attenuate the enhancing effect of post-training epinephrine on retention of an inhibitory avoidance response', *Behavioural Brain Research* 9 (1983), 49–58.

32. Packard, M. G., Introini-Collison, I. and McGaugh, J. L., 'Stria terminalis lesions attenuate memory enhancement produced by intracaudate nucleus injections of oxotremorine', *Neurobiology of Learning and Memory* 65 (1996), 278–82.

33. Roozendaal B., 'Glucocorticoids and the regulation of memory consolidation', *Psychoneuroendocrinology* 25 (2000), 213–38; Sandi, C., and Rose, S. P. R., 'Corticosterone enhances long-term retention in one-day-old chicks trained in a weak passive avoidance learning paradigm', *Brain Research* 647 (1994), 106–112.

34. McEwen, B. S., 'The neurobiology of stress: from serendipity to clinical relevance', *Brain Research* 886 (2000), 172–89.

35. McGaugh, J. L. and Roozendaal, B., 'Role of adrenal stress hormones in forming lasting memories in the brain', *Current Opinion in Neurobiology* 12 (2002), 205–10.

36. DeQuervain, D. J.-F., Roozendaal, B. and McGaugh, J. L., 'Stress and glucocorticoids impair retrieval of long-term spatial memory', *Nature* 394 (1998), 787–90; de Quervain, D. J.-F., Roozendaal, B., Nitsch, R. M., McGaugh, J. L. and Hock, C., 'Acute cortisone administration impairs retrieval of long-term declarative memory in healthy subjects', *Nature Neuroscience* 3 (2000), 313–14.

37. Cahill, L., Prins, B., Weber, M. and McGaugh, J. L., 'β-adrenergic activation and memory for emotional events', *Nature* 371 (1994), 702–4.

38. Reist, C., Duffy, J. G., Fujimoto, K. and Cahill, L., 'Beta-adrenergic blockade and emotional memory in PTSD', *International Journal of Neuropsychopharmacology* 4 (2001), 377–83; O'Carroll, R. E., Drysdale, E., Cahill, L., Shajahan, P., and Ebmeier, K. P., 'Stimulation of the noradrenergic system enhances and blockade reduces memory

for emotional material in man', *Psychological Medicine* 29 (1999), 1083–88; Southwick, S. M., Davis, M., Horner, B., Cahill, L., Morgan, C. A., Gold, P. E., Bremner, J. D. and Charney, D. C., 'Relationship of enhanced norepinephrine activity during memory consolidation to enhanced long-term memory in humans', *American Journal of Psychiatry* 159 (2002), 1420–22.

39. Nielson, K. A. and Jensen, R. A., 'Beta-adrenergic receptor antagonist antihypertensive medications impair arousal-induced modulation of working memory in elderly humans', *Behavioral and Neural Biology* 62 (1995), 190–200.

40. Jensen, R. A., 'Neural pathways mediating the modulation of learning and memory by arousal', in Gold, P. E. and Greenough, W. T. (eds.), *Memory Consolidation: Essays in Honor of James L. McGaugh*, American Psychological Association, Washington, D. C., 2001, pp. 129–40.

41. Gold, P. E., 'A proposed neurobiological basis for regulating memory storage for significant events', in Winograd, E. and Neisser, U. (eds.), *Affect and Accuracy in Recall: Studies of 'Flashbulb' Memories*, Cambridge University Press, New York, 1992, pp. 141–61; Gold, P. E., and Stone, W. S., 'Neuroendocrine factors in age-related memory dysfunctions: Studies in animals and humans', *Neurobiology of Aging* 9 (1988), 709–17; Korol, D. L. and Gold, P. E., 'Glucose, memory and aging', *American Journal of Clinical Nutrition* 67 (1998), 764S–771S.

42. Buchanan, T. W., and Lovallo, W. R., 'Enhanced memory for emotional material following stress-level cortisol treatment in humans', *Psychoneuroendocrinology* 26 (2001), 307–17.

43. Schelling, G., 'Effects of stress hormones on traumatic memory formation and the development of posttraumatic stress disorder in critcally ill patients', *Neurobiology of Learning and Memory*, 78 (2002), 596–609.

44. Cahill, L., Babinsky, R., Markowitsch, H. J. and McGaugh, J. L., 'The amygdala and emotional memory', *Nature* 377 (1995), 295–6; Adolphs, R., Cahill, L., Schul, R. and Babinsky, R., 'Impaired declarative memory for emotional stimuli following bilateral amygdala damage in humans', *Learning and Memory* 4 (1997), 291–300.

45. Phelps, E. A. and Anderson, A. K., 'Emotional memory: What does the amygdala do?', *Current Biology* 7 (1997), R311–R314; LaBar, K. S. and Phelps, E. A., 'Arousal-mediated memory consolidation: Role of the medial temporal lobe in humans', *Psychological Sciences* 9 (1998), 490–93.

46. Hamann, S. B., Cahill, L., McGaugh, J. L., Squire, L. R., 'Intact

enhancement of declarative memory for emotional material in amnesia', *Learning and Memory* 4 (1997), 301–9; Moayeri, S., Cahill, L., Jin, Y. and Potkin, S. G., 'Relative sparing of emotionally influenced memory in Alzheimer's disease', *Neuroreport* 11 (2000), 653–5; Kazui, H., Mori, E., Hashimoto, M., Hirono, N., Imamura, T., Tanimukai, S., Hanihara, T. and Cahill, L., 'Impact of emotion on memory', *British Journal of Psychiatry* 177 (2000), 343–7.

47. Cahill, L., Haier, R. J., Fallon, J., Alkire, M., Tang, C., Keator, D., Wu, J. and McGaugh, J. L., 'Amygdala activity at encoding correlated with long-term, free recall of emotional information', *Proceedings, National Academy of Sciences, USA* 93 (1996), 8016–21.

48. Cahill, L., Haier, R. J., White, N. S., Fallon, J., Kilpatrick, L., Lawrence, C., Potkin, S. G., and Alkire, M. T., 'Sex-related difference in amygdala activity during emotionally influenced memory storage', *Neurobiology of Learning and Memory* 75 (2001), 1–9.

49. Hamann, S. G., Elt, T., Grafton, S., and Kilts, C., 'Amygdala activity related to enhanced memory for pleasant and aversive stimuli', *Nature Neuroscience* 2 (1999), 289–93.

50. Canli, T., Zhao, Z., Brewer, J., Gabrieli, J. D. and Cahill, L., 'Event related activation in the human amygdala associates with later memory for individual emotional experience', *Journal of Neuroscience* 20 (2000), RC99.

51. Mori, E., Ikeda, M., Hirono, N., Kitagaki, H., Imamura, T. and Shimomura, T., 'Amygdalar volume and emotional memory in Alzheimer's disease', *American Journal of Psychiatry* 156 (1999), 216–22.

52. LeDoux, J., 'The amygdala and emotion: a view through fear', in Aggleton, J. P. (ed.), *The Amygdala: A Functional Analysis*, Oxford University Press, London, 2000, pp. 289–310.

53. Davis, M., 'The role of the amygdala in conditioned and unconditioned fear and anxiety', in Aggleton, J. P. (ed.), *The Amygdala: A Functional Analysis*, Oxford University Press, London, 2000, pp. 213–88.

54. Cahill, L., Vazdarjanova, A. and Setlow, B., 'The basolateral amygdala complex is involved with, but is not necessary for, rapid acquisition of Pavlovian "fear" conditioning', *European Journal of Neuroscience* 12 (2000), 3044–50; Killcross, S., Robbins, T. W., and Everitt, B. J., 'Different types of fear-conditioned behaviour mediated by separate nuclei within amygdala', *Nature* 388 (1997), 377–80; Vazdarjanova, A. and McGaugh, J. L., 'Basolateral amygdala is not a critical locus for memory of contextual fear conditioning', *Proceedings, National Academy of Sciences, USA* 95 (1998), 15003–7; Lehmann, H., Treit,

D., and Parent, M. B., 'Amygdala lesions do not impair shock-probe avoidance retention performance', *Behavioral Neuroscience* 114 (2000), 107–16.

55. Cahill, L., and McGaugh, J. L., 'Mechanisms of emotional arousal and lasting declarative memory', *Trends in Neuroscience* 21 (1998), 294–9; McGaugh, J. L., 'Memory consolidation and the amygdala: a systems perspective', *Trends in Neurosciences* 25 (2002), 456–61; McGaugh, J. L., 'The amygdala regulates memory consolidation', in Squire, L. R. and Schacter, D. L. (eds.) *Neuropsychology of Memory, 3rd Edition*, The Guilford Press, New York, 2002, pp. 437–49.

56. Bliss, T. V. P. and Lomo, T., Long-lasting potentiation of synaptic transmission in the dentate gyrus of the anaesthetized rabbit following stimulation of the perforant path', *Journal of Physiology* 232 (1973), 331–56.

57. Ikegaya, Y., Saito, H. and Abe, K., 'Requirement of basolateral amygdale neuron activity for the induction of long-term potentiation in the dentate gyrus *in vivo*', *Brain Research* 67 (1995), 351–4.

58. Martin, S. J., Grimwood, S. J. and Morris, R. G. M., 'Synaptic plasticity and memory: and evaluation of the hypothesis', *Annual Review of Neuroscience* 23 (2000), 649–711.

59. Schafe, G. E., Nader, K., Blair, H. T., LeDoux, J. E., 'Memory consolidation of Pavlovian fear conditioning: a cellular and molecular perspective', *Trends in Neuroscience* 24 (2001), 540–46.

60. Squire, L. R. and Alvarez, P., 'Retrograde amnesia and memory consolidation: a neurobiological perspective', *Current Opinion in Neurobiology* 5 (1995), 169–177; Teyler, T. J. and DiScenna, P., 'The hippocampal memory indexing theory', *Behavioral Neuroscience* 100 (1986), 147–54; McClelland, J. L., McNaughton, B. L., and O'Reilly, R. C., 'Why there are complementary learning systems in the hippocampus and neocortex: insights from the successes and failures of connectionist models of learning and memory', *Psychological Review* 102 (1995), 419–57.

Chapter 6: Meandering and Monumental Memory

1. Tulving, E., *Elements of Episodic Memory*, Oxford University Press, New York, 1983.

2. Bartlett, F. C., *Remembering*, Cambridge University Press, Cambridge, 1932.

3. Bartlett, p. 65.

4. Bartlett, p. 75.

5. Schmolck, H., Buffalo, E. A. and Squire, L. R. (2000).

6. Deese, J., 'On the prediction of occurrence of particular verbal intrusions in immediate recall', *Journal of Experimental Psychology* 58 (1959), 17–22.

7. Roediger, H. L. III and McDermott, K. B., 'Creating false memories. Remembering words not presented in lists', *Journal of Experimental Psychology: Learning, Memory and Cognition* 21 (1995), 803–14.

8. Loftus, E. F., Feldman, J. and Dashiell, R., 'The reality of illusory memories', in Schacter, D. L. (ed.), *Memory Distortion*, Harvard University Press, 1995, pp. 47–68.

9. Loftus et al., p. 63.

10. Loftus et al., p. 63.

11. Ceci, S. J., False beliefs: Some developmental and clinical consideration', in Schacter, D. L. (ed.), *Memory Distortion*, Harvard University Press, 1995, pp. 91–125.

12. Ceci, p. 102.

13. Loftus, E. and Ketcham, K., *The Myth of Repressed Memory*, St Martin's, Griffin, New York, 1994, p. 38.

14. Pitman, R. K. and Orr, S. P., 'Psychophysiology of emotional memory networks in posttraumatic stress disorder', in McGaugh, J. L., Weinberger, N. M. and Lynch, G. (eds.), *Brain and Memory: Modulation and Mediation of Neuroplasticity*, Oxford University Press, New York, 1995, pp. 75–83.

15. Pitman and Orr (1995), p. 80.

16. Pitman and Orr (1995), pp. 77–8.

17. Pitman and Orr, p. 81.

18. Pitman, R. K., Sanders, K. M., Zusman, R. M., Healy, A. R., Cheema, F., Lasko, N. B., Cahill, L. and Orr, S. P., 'Pilot study of secondary prevention of posttraumatic stress disorder with propanolol', *Biological Psychiatry* 51 (2002), 189–92. Also see Fletcher, T. and Cahill, L. 'Propranolol for reemergent posttraumatic stress disorder following an event of retraumatization: a case study', *Journal of Traumatic Stress* 15 (2002), 433–37. Treatment with propranolol rapidly and markedly reduced symptoms of PTSD in a patient who had experienced a series of automobile accidents.

19. Vaiva, G., Ducrocq, F., Jezequel, K., Averland, B., Lestavel, P., Brunet, A., Marmar, C. R., 'Peritraumatic prescription of propranolol decreases acute PTSD symptoms', International Society for Traumatic Stress Studies (ISTSS), Baltimore, November 2002.

20. James, W. (1890), p. 680.

21. Borges, J. L., *Labyrinths, Selected short Stories and Other Writings*, Introduction by André Maurois. Edited by James Irby and Donald

Yates. 38 'fictions', essays and parables. New Directions Publishing Company, 1962, pp. 59–66.

22. Borges (1962), pp. 63–6.
23. Luria, A. R., *A Little Book about a Vast Memory: The Mind of a Mnemonist*, Harvard University Press, 1968.
24. Luria, p. 61.
25. Luria, p. 28.
26. Luria, p. 159.
27. Hunt, E., and Love, T., 'How good can memory be?', in Melton, A. W., and Martin, E. (eds.), *Coding Processes in Human Memory*, Winston-Wiley, 1972, pp. 237–60.
28. Hunt and Love, pp. 259–60.
29. Hurst, L. C. and Mulhall, D. J., 'Another calendar savant', *British Journal of Psychiatry* 152 (1988), 274–7.
30. Heavey, L., Ping, L. and Hermelin, B., 'A date to remember: The nature of memory in savant calendrical calculators', *Psychological Medicine* 29 (1999), 145–60.
31. Howe, M. J. A. and Smith, J., 'Calendar calculating in "idiot savants": How do they do it?', *British Journal of Psychology* 79 (1988), 371–86.
32. O'Conner, N. and Hermelin, B., 'Idiot savant calendrical calculators: maths or memory?', *Psychological Medicine* 14 (1984), 801–6.
33. Lester, D., 'Idiot savants: a review', *Psychology* 14 (1977), 20–23.

Chapter 7: Memorabilia: Summing Up

1. James, W. (1890).
2. Pavlov, I. P. (1927).
3. Thorndike, E. L. (1898).
4. Tolman, E. C. (1932).
5. Hebb, D. O. (1949).
6. Duncan, C. P. (1949), Müller, G. E. and Pilzecker, A. (1990).
7. McGaugh, J. L. (1973).
8. McGaugh, J. L. (2002).
9. Pitman, R. K. and Orr, S. P. (1995).
10. Bartlett, F. C. (1932).
11. Loftus, E. F., Feldman, J. and Dashiell, R., 1995.
12. Borges, J. L. (1962), pp. 59–66.
13. Luria, A. R. (1968).
14. Schacter, Daniel L., *The Seven Sins of Memory*, Houghton Mifflin Company, Boston, 2001; Eichenbaum, H. and Cohen, N. J., *From Conditioning to Conscious Recollection: Memory Systems of the Brain*, Oxford University Press, New York, 2001; Bourtchouladze, R.,

Memories are Made of This, Weidenfield and Nicolson, London, 2002; Squire, Larry R., and Kandel, E. R., *Memory From Mind to Molecules*, Scientific American Library, New York, 1999; Dudai, Y., *Memory from A to Z*, Oxford University Press, Oxford, 2002.

Index